Intermittent Moving

How I lost my pants and mastered my weight

Move more • Sit less • Master your weight

Barbara & Kevin Kunz

Published by RTS Publishing, New Mexico, USA

ISBN 9781686640445

Produced by **Bookworx**
Designer Peggy Sadler
Proofreader Jill Schneider

Books by Barbara and Kevin Kunz
The Complete Guide to Foot Reflexology (Third Edition), RRP Press, 2005
Reflexology, Health at your fingertips, Dorling Kindersley, 2003
Complete Reflexology for Life, Dorling Kindersley, 2007
Un-Sit Your Life: Change your sitting habits, Empower your life, RTS Press, 2015

Contents

About the authors

We are reflexologists, researchers and authors of 24 reflexology books published in 24 languages. We have enjoyed a lifelong study of reflexology, the reflex actions influencing the body and health, prompted as pressure is applied to the feet and hands in a systematic and targeted approach.

It was a newspaper article that drew our interest to sitting too much. We saw the reported resulting health problems as happening when not enough pressure is applied to the feet as one sits too much and walks too little. Researching the data was fascinating, but just as with reflexology we applied the concepts to our own lives. We "un-sat" our lives. For Kevin the results were especially dramatic with a weight loss of 60 pounds. For both of us, we've shaped up and become more energetic.

OUR MISSION

We won't sit still any longer for unnatural weight gain and ill health. We hope you won't either.

Take a stand. Move a little to get closer to your goal of losing weight while gaining a healthier life style. To further such goals we created a system of intermittent moving, timing your sit-stand-move time to master your weight naturally and successfully. Breaking the habit of sitting can change your life and put you in control.

Don't just sit there. Go for it.

Part one

INTERMITTENT MOVING

Move more, sit less, master your weight

1 Introduction: mastering your weight

Something is missing in our quest to control our weight. Great diets don't always work. Fantastic exercise programs don't always help.

Starving yourself often seems to have a reverse effect. What if there was something so simple you could do and it would make all the difference to your weight and waistline? Would you do it?

What if there's a way to control your appetite that doesn't require pills or surgery or extreme diets? Would you do it? What if, in addition, it is free, requires no equipment, isn't strenuous and can be done anywhere and at any time? Would you do it?

You can become the master of your weight and health. You can literally take the steps necessary to change and design the body you want.

What would you do to get back in control? Instead of avoiding the mirror, you would look for mirrors. Instead of making excuses for your weight, there is no need for excuses to be made. Instead of the sense of isolation, frustration, anxiety and feeling all alone, you feel positive about where you're going.

All this sounds too good to be true. But it's not. You can become the master of your weight and health. You can literally take the steps necessary to change and design the body you want.

It could be a lot simpler than you think. It's all about moving more and sitting less, moving mountains by moving often, leaving your chair and moving for short periods throughout the day. Small is beautiful. Small efforts at moving are beautiful because you can achieve more of your goal with less strenuous patterns of exercise.

This book is about intermittent moving: timing how often you move during the day and evening so your metabolism doesn't stall. It's this lack of movement that contributes to weight and waistline. Our goal is to show you how you can time your sit-stand-move time to manipulate your weight naturally and successfully.

Weight loss happened for me; it can happen for you

Kevin's Story

I felt like I would never change. I was stuck with the weight I was. I was stuck with the waistline I had. Then I lost six inches off my waistline and just over 40 pounds in a year. Almost four years later and it's still gone. I've lost more weight and waistline.

I didn't change my eating habits. I didn't exercise more. After all, neither had helped before. It even seemed like dieting was counter-productive. Whatever I lost, I'd gain back and then some.

What happened to change my life? I became interested in my wife's research about the health perils of prolonged sitting. In response, I created a standing desk for work hours and a standing platform to hold my iPad during the evening. Underfoot where I stood were mats with raised textured surfaces—reflexology mats.

It occurred to me that not-sitting was having a profound effect on my waistline and weight.

As time passed, the unexpected happened. My pants were looser. One day they slipped off—as I was standing in my driveway (apologies to my neighbors). It occurred to me that not-sitting was having a profound effect on my waistline and weight. I wanted to do more and I did.

Most curious, I felt like I was shaping up—from the inside out. Not only is my waistline reduced, it's firmed up. I'm seeing abdominal muscles instead of flab. It's magic to someone who had tried almost everything to no effect.

Then there's the reduction in my appetite. Before, if I had food in front of me, I'd eat it with no stopping. Now I actually feel full and stop eating.

Every time I tell this story to someone who, like me, has struggled to lose weight, it strikes a chord with them and I hear: "That's the way I feel. I've tried everything—I even flunked out of Jenny Craig!"

Then I tell them about what sitting too much does to the body, how our bodies are not designed for it and how it dis-regulates the metabolism of the body and mechanisms important to maintaining weight—among other things.

And, it suddenly makes sense to them—why their efforts to keep weight off are doomed to failure. The difference in my life was the thing we haven't been told. It was a very simple fact that made all the difference: we can't sit still. We shouldn't sit still.

It was all about moving and it was all about timing the moving. Why didn't I know? Why wasn't I told?

Why is this important? Moving is the mechanism of our metabolisms. How much and how often we sit and stand and move directly affects our metabolisms. We don't even think about sitting and standing and moving. And we don't really think how these simple things impact our metabolisms. I certainly didn't. Once I knew about the importance of timing my sit-stand-move habits, it was the magic trick that flipped the switch on my weight loss. Suddenly, things started happening.

I discovered the importance of moving the right amount of time to lose and maintain my weight loss.

You can too.

2 The importance of moving

For many of us, weight is a lifelong cross to bear. Being overweight is the feeling that nothing will ever change. No matter what you do. No matter what you try.

Your weight problem not only seems to continue but it gets worse, no matter what you do, what diet your try or how much exercise you do.

It impacts all kinds of things, particularly your own self-esteem. Can this endless crawl towards a bigger and bigger you be stopped?

Yes, it can but only if you understand why it's happening. There's something simple triggering it and with the right knowledge you can stop it and reverse it.

There's no magic to it. No magic diets. No magic exercise programs. And, best of all, it's free.

It worked for me. I don't think about gaining weight any more. I would like to lose more weight but it's not the act of desperation it once was. I am in control.

There's no magic to it. No magic diets. No magic exercise programs. And, best of all, it's free.

There is hope and the hope comes from research and proven methods of harnessing the body's own ability to maintain weight. It's about matching what you do throughout your day, with your body's own natural rhythms of moving. Meet your body's needs to move and you'll unlock the path to weight loss and control.

That's what this book is about. It's about learning simple principles that will change the trajectory of your weight and put you in control.

Your body needs to move

Your body has incredible capabilities. What is holding you back? What's keeping you from achieving your absolute best potential? You haven't been told, you haven't been given the opportunity to do what needs to be done. There are fundamentals of life. We need water. We need oxygen. We need food. Without these elements, we cease to survive, much less thrive.

Here's a simple secret: your body needs to move. Just as it needs oxygen to breathe and food to eat. Your body needs to get up and move. We eat food every day. We breathe oxygen constantly.

Your body needs to move. Just as it needs oxygen to breathe and food to eat.

Movement is critical. Just as food nourishes the body, so too does moving. Just as periods without food create problems, so too do long periods without moving. It your body is to perform at its best, it needs the nourishment of moving. And moving is not exercise.

We've all become aware of the need to focus on proper nutrition, focus on exercise. Focus on drinking enough water. Focus on breathing properly. None of these deals with a basic fact: the background tone of our bodies is determined by every step taken, every moment spent sitting. Focus on moving is perhaps the final frontier in maintaining our bodies.

You want a better life, it's time to move, but first, consider why you may not be moving enough.

The blame game

You hit this wall and the wall says you're eating too much and you're not exercising. And, you stall in that position. You try all kinds of diets, exercise to the extreme. You try a little bit and then you gradually just stop.

You can blame weight gain on calories consumed. You can blame it on not exercising. You can blame it on a family history of weight problems. Sure, all of these play a factor. But, there is more.

The big picture is moving. If you're not moving enough your metabolism slows. If you're not getting up and moving, your body's natural appetite controls go awry. You feel hungry all the time and you don't stop eating when you should.

Moving is magical. It can put you in shape and whittle away at your waistline. It can help your cardiovascular system to work better. It can fire up your brain, help you focus and fight dementia. Moving feeds your brain the oxygen and nutrients it needs to function at its best. Cognitive reserve is the big idea that it's possible to protect yourself from brain deterioration. Do you have cognitive reserve?

Trained to sit

When you think about it, dogs aren't the only ones trained to sit. There are pressures that tell us to sit down and sit still. Being immobile is considered a good thing.

From an early age we're encouraged and, yes, even trained to sit.

From an early age we're encouraged and, yes, even trained to sit. Did you ever hear your mother say, "Sit still and be good and don't bother your mom!". Sit still in class. Sit at your desk or workstation and do your work. Sit in meetings. Then there's transportation—still in the car, on the bus, on the train, in the plane. We place a high social premium in sitting still.

Altogether, that's hours of **required** sitting a day. Whether by encouragement or necessity, sitting is dictated by society's standards, not by our bodies' needs. Then there's the entertainment factor. We are enticed to sit to be entertained. The television, the computer screen, the game playing device or the cell phone—all of them call to us to have a seat and enjoy. It's really faux movement, with activity happening in your head but not to your body.

Either way you're still impacting your body, how it operates and how much you weigh. Get ready to take a stand. Become a movement maverick.

Breaking the sitting habit

You, like all of us, have been brainwashed by society to think sitting is good. Sitting quietly is polite. Sitting still is mature. Yes, sitting is restful and you need rest but more isn't necessarily better. There's a healthy balance between how long you sit, how often you get up and how much you move.

The real measure of sitting is when you realize that you haven't moved in quite a while. You've been sitting too long. According to researchers, if you've sat an hour, you've sat too long.

According to researchers, if you've sat an hour, you've sat too long.

Sitting is equated with good things: with good behavior in school, being productive at work, being relaxed at home. It's a hard nut to crack, moving when you've spent a lifetime learning to sit still. It's going to take commitment to break this habit. Moving is a form of low intensity exercise. You get into an alliance with your body. It's getting into a rhythm. I'm not asking you to go to the extremes; I'm just asking you to do intermittent, low effort, simple changes.

It's ok to be on a diet. Why not go on another kind of diet, one your body and weight will appreciate? One that will make for a healthy environment for your mood and future? One that actually produces the results that you want?

Easiest "diet" ever

This is one of the easiest diets ever. It's easiest because it's easy to do. As you'll see below, if you stand up and move, you will change your metabolism. And that will change your body.

Yet, it's one of the hardest things to do. The hard part is doing it consistently enough so that your body is conditioned into its new way of being.

Let's be honest: we all like to sit. You sit; you sit; you sit. And, all the while, your body is building up not just weight but risk factors for illness and disease.

We humans have a tendency to make things comfortable. We literally get stuck; we get static; we don't move. It's like an old car sitting there. It's fully capable of moving but if it sits there too long, it no longer has the capability of moving.

Here's your motivation: getting up and moving can give you the ability to lose weight and waistline.

Getting up and moving can give you the ability to lose weight and waistline.

What if you could free yourself from all the time you spend thinking about and adjusting your life to your weight? What if you could improve your quality of life? You might also extend your life. You can save money not being ill, losing time at work or paying co-pays for doctor visits. Do it for yourself. Do it for your loved ones.

In a nutshell: you lose weight, you lose waistline. You have better health, more energy. It's free. It's easy to do. It's much less strenuous than most exercise programs. No learning curve. No heavy equipment.

Start moving. Start losing.

We'll guide you through ideas to add movement to your day and evening and help you overcome impediments to moving.

3 Getting your body to help you lose weight

Yes, it's that simple. Stand and move frequently enough and weight mastery happens.

You're fighting to lose weight. You've cut back on calories. You go to the gym. Weight gain continues. But it seems your body's not listening. What's going on? While you're busy watching your weight, so too is your body. That's right, parts of your body serve as weight watchers.

And because of this, your body can help you lose weight. You just have to ask it the right way.

Yes, there are parts of your body glad to be of help. To enlist this help you just have to stand up and move. Every footstep puts into action your mind and your mind will help your body.

Maybe you're not sending your body the right messages by the actions you take:
- When you stand up, you activate parts of your metabolism specifically associated with weight and obesity.
- When you stand up your body's automatic

While you're busy watching your weight, so too is your body. That's right, parts of your body serve as weight watchers.

appetite controls go to work helping adjust whether or not you feel hungry and need to eat.

- When you don't stand up for long periods of time, when you have been sitting too long, your body literally turns down your metabolism and other systems. This seems counter-intuitive but this is why it's important to move more and sit less.

Your body's metabolism re-set as you move
Kevin's Story

It takes 90 seconds to activate your metabolism as you stand up and move. This is not a secret weight loss formula. This is fact. 90 seconds and I can activate my metabolism? This was a really striking fact to me.

Metabolism is all about feeding our bodies the nutrients we need. Your metabolism goes to work as muscles "ask" for nutrition.

Every step you take puts to work the parts of your body important to your metabolism and weight.

Muscles "ask" for nutrients as we stand and, especially, walk. The nutrients are fats and sugar circulating in the blood stream.

Every step you take puts to work the parts of your body important to your metabolism and weight. The muscles that move you forward? They are part of the "fat vacuuming" system set to draw fat from your blood stream into the muscles as they move. Also being drawn from the blood stream as muscles move is blood sugar. This is your metabolism being re-set.

FIGHT GRAVITY

You need to fight gravity by standing and moving a certain amount of the day, every day. Think of fighting gravity as your personal invisible gym. Every time you move and stimulate your muscles, you are in your gym. You are renewing your body. You are winning your fight with gravity.

BIOMARKERS

"Good" cholesterol, triglycerides and blood sugar levels are biomarkers associated with weight obesity. Other important biomarkers are blood pressure and leptin levels. Leptin is important in regulating your appetite or telling your body you are hungry.

Leg muscles don't move as one sits. Sit too long and the metabolism slows. This happens because sitting is seen by the body as an activity with little need for nutrition. Without the need for nutrients, the absorption of the fats and sugar that fuel movement also slows down. The result can only be described as disarray.

This disarray is marked by abnormal levels of fats such as triglycerides and "good" cholesterol and glucose or blood sugar. These abnormal levels are associated with weight and obesity. Researcher Dr. James Levine of the Mayo Clinic explains this link between standing and metabolism: "… within 90 seconds of standing up, the muscular and cellular systems that process blood sugar, triglycerides, and cholesterol—which are mediated by insulin—are activated." In other words within 90 seconds of standing up, your metabolism goes to work.

Furthermore, if you have been sitting an hour, "… the cellular mechanisms involved in the maintenance of your body and health are shutting down." Your metabolism slows as it is being thrown into disarray. Your weight and other key health factors are being impacted.

Appetite under control—or not?
Kevin's story

It used to be I tried to be not hungry. That didn't work. Then I thought there was a magic place I could go where I wouldn't feel hungry. I wanted to be in that place where I would spontaneously feel full and just stop eating. Then I found that place. Once I started to move more, my appetite began to take care of itself. I had finally found that place where I could eat, feel satisfied and then be ready to stop eating. That was the place.

How do we know we're full and don't need to eat more? This is a key component in gaining or losing weight.

How do we know we're full and don't need to eat more? This is a key component in gaining or losing weight. Our body signals us when we are full and to stop eating or when we are not and to continue on. This appetite control is in your control.

Sitting too much and not moving enough sets off a chain of events that throws the body's natural appetite out of whack. The result is eating more food than necessary. You start to consume more than you need to move through your day, you start to gain weight.

Metabolic appetite control

As our metabolisms function, our appetite controls are turned on. As we walk or stand, muscles begin to take up sugar and fats from the blood stream to be used as fuel. At the same time, circulating in the blood stream are indicators of "fuel use." The hormone insulin, is an indicator of how much blood sugar is in the blood stream and available for the muscles to use. The hormone leptin serves the same purpose only it indicates the available fat. As your blood circulates through your body, carrying the leptin and insulin, it passes into the part of the brain that is responsible for controlling the appetite. This part of the brain, the hypothalamus, acts to regulate other hormones that are related to triggering feelings of fullness in the stomach and the intestines. Once the hypothalamus receives information about fat and sugar levels in the body, the "switch" is thrown and your body will begin to increase or dampen your appetite and your desire to eat or stop eating.

This appetite control system can be thrown into disarray when the muscles do not move often enough. Sugar remains in the blood stream instead of being "vacuumed "up by the muscles. Leptin levels also increase. What follows is a sort of mild metabolic chaos: the muscles are perceived as resisting the "uptake" of glucose or blood sugar. This is known as "insulin resistance". Similarly the increased amounts of unused leptin are perceived by the body as "leptin resistance." Your appetite controls begin to receive faulty messages. Your appetite controls go awry. You get "falsely" hungry. You eat more than you require.

This appetite control system can be thrown into disarray when the muscles do not move often enough.

The leg bones connected to appetite control

Who knew that the long bones in your legs would have anything to do with your appetite control? According to researcher Dr John-Olov Jansson of the University of Gothenburg, when you stand and move, cells in the bones "sense changes in body mass and then somehow, (this part is unknown to science,) initiate alterations to appetite and eating that then can return the body to its previous weight". It's hard to decide whether that information is as surprising as the part that it is known and yet unexplained by science.

Thus when we stand, the bone cells in the legs send messages about how much weight the bones are bearing. When we sit, no messages are sent. More sitting leads to fewer opportunities for the bone cells to do their part in sensing weight. The weight that they determine as we stand, go into the body's calculation of how much we weigh and if that weight has changed. Based on that information, our appetite is triggered or dampened and our eating patterns are set.

Who knew that the long bones in your legs would have anything to do with your appetite control?

Dr. Jansson also notes "The possibility (of cells in the long bones helping to determine appetite) could help to explain why sitting for hours is associated with obesity…" He goes onto note "When we sit much of our body is supported by cushions rather than bones, leaving our skeletons unaware of how much we actually weigh and whether that amount has changed or should change."(Reynolds, Gretchen, "How Our Bones Might Help Keep Our Weight in Check," *New York Times*, Jan. 17, 2018).

The take away—extended sitting stops the long bones of the legs from their job as serving as a trigger to appetite control.

Overfed fat cells, inflammation and weight challenges

Those who are overweight are more likely to have elevated indicators of chronic, low-grade inflammation or infection. There may not be an actual infection in the body. However, elevated indicators are also tied to uninterrupted and length periods of sitting.

Inflammation is measured by the level of C-reactive protein or CRP. These level increase as weight increases. As weight decreases, the CRP also decreases.

Why would this be? It has to do with those pesky fat cells. Fat cells store fat. Fat cells respond to a high calorie diet by storing more fat. Overfed fat cells respond by creating the same chemical reaction they would if they encountered bacteria or viruses. The immune system responds as if there is an infection and begins an inflammatory response.

The more you sit, the higher levels of CRP are found in your body. Four hours a day of sitting in front of a screen such as a

BE MINDFUL

Mindfulness—as you get up and move, remember the long bones of your legs are communicating important weight information to other parts of your body. This information is helping trigger your appetite control and your weight loss efforts. This won't happen if you do not let the leg bones move you around.

computer after work, can translate into high levels of CRP. In a study done by British researcher Dr. Emmanuel Stamatakis, participants in the study who sat for four hours had double the amount of normal CRP as those who only sat for two hours. Participants who sat at home for more than six hours a day had CRP levels three times as high as the two-hour sitters.

Your take away: sitting time impacts a body measure associated with weight.

THE RISKS OF ELEVATED CRP

Elevated CPR levels are also associated with cardiovascular disease, cancer and other lifestyle conditions. Inflammation can play a role in hardening of the arteries, (atherosclerosis). This condition is known to cause at least 50 percent of all strokes. Four hours or more of sitting at home in the evening, more than doubles the risk of heart attack and stroke, according to the Stamatakis study, noted above.

Summary—why not moving contributes to your weight gain

Our bodies and our metabolisms are designed to stand and move about most of the time. We are not designed to sit most of the time. Yet we do. Sitting is seen by the body as an activity that requires little nutrition. This signals the metabolism to slow down. Chaos follows. Your body begins to function inappropriately. Gaining weight is the outcome.

It's all about the metabolism. It's all about the calories. It is related to modern life. Sitting and not moving around has taken the place of those activities that expend calories. We are no longer hunters and gatherers. Few of us are farmers or wandering nomads.

This impacts our appetite control. Sit too much and move too little and our appetite control system is thrown off. But how much sitting does it take to disrupt the metabolic and appetitive control systems?

Your metabolism slows down ninety percent after just thirty minutes of sitting. This will impact the measures of metabolism, the fat and sugar levels. The levels of the "fat vacuuming" enzyme drops by 90–95 percent after a day spent sitting.

One day of sitting reduces insulin action by 39 percent. Thus, the body's ability to measure and control the appetite mechanism is thrown off as well.

METABOLISM IN DISARRAY

Weight gain is a risk associated with the metabolism in disarray. Diabetes, cardiovascular disease, autoimmune disorders dementia and Alzheimer 's disease are also risks associated with this type of metabolic dysfunction.

DIABETES
• Nine percent of Americans are diabetic.
• Thirty percent of overweight people are diabetic.
• Eighty percent of diabetics are overweight.
The common factor in these statistics is sugar left circulating in the blood stream due to too much inactivity. The body misinterprets this excess sugar as a need to produce more insulin. But more insulin isn't really needed and the muscles resist taking it up.

Insulin resistance occurs. There is a kind of chaos in the sugar—muscle need—insulin production. Eventually the pancreas solves the problem by not producing sufficient

METABOLISM IN DISARRAY continued

insulin and Type II diabetes is the likely outcome. Risk indicators for diabetes include impaired metabolism of sugars, or insulin resistance and increased weight around the middle. Both of these are influenced by prolonged sitting. All of these impact how much you weigh.

CARDIOVASCULAR DISEASE

Sitting too much and moving too little affects fat storage and fat use. Fat is not taken up to fuel muscles on the move. Instead, it is stored in fat cells or in the walls of arteries. This sets the stage for a multitude of possible cardiovascular problems, such as stroke, heart attack and vascular disease.

AUTOIMMUNE DISORDERS

Inflammation fires up your immune system. The immune system responds as if it had an invader to fight. Chronic inflammation is the immune system on high alert with no rest, no resolution. Eventually the immune system begins to attack healthy tissue. The body is attacking itself. This is the picture of an autoimmune disease. These have proliferated right along with our sedentary life style. Thirty-two percent of Americans have elevated levels of CRP. Fifty percent of overweight Americans have elevated levels of this inflammation indicator. Seventy five percent of obese people show elevated levels of CRP.

DEMENTIA AND ALZHEIMER'S DISEASE

Science has been hard pressed to identify exactly why we are plagued by dementia and Alzheimer's disease. What is known

METABOLISM IN DISARRAY continued

is that metabolism plays a role. Cognitive decline is part of both dementia and Alzheimer's disease. One study reported by CBS news showed that those in middle age who had two or more metabolic risk factors such as abnormal triglyceride levels, very high cholesterol readings, elevated blood glucose levels, high blood pressure or waistlines above 42 inches, would have poorer cognitive functioning ten years later. People with normal weight face fewer possibility for cognitive decline in old age than those who are obese, obese and healthy or those with metabolism disorders.

Help your body help you to lose weight

Help your body help you. Moving more each day helps your body re-set your metabolism, which will reset biomarkers that are important to controlling you appestat and therefore your weight.

Change your metabolism by engaging in activities that engage your body's metabolism and other functions. By engaging and changing the function of your body, you help your body work better, alleviating the health risks created by prolonged sitting. It's really not as complex as it sounds.

Read on to find out how.

4 Change your lifestyle, change your weight

It is said that a journey of 1,000 miles starts with a single footstep. A new habit starts with the triggering of a single action or activity.

A habit is pattern of behavior acquired through frequent repetition. And so it is with your sitting habit. To be successful in triggering weight loss: you want to interrupt sitting and you want to do it frequently and consistently.

When you truly enjoy success in forming an intermittent moving habit that helps your body, you just get up and move. You don't really think about it.

Moving through the day takes on a new meaning. You realize that every movement has a positive reaction from your body. It is the accumulation of these tens and hundreds and thousands of muscle actions creating little movements throughout the day that will contribute to your weight loss efforts.

To be successful in triggering weight loss: you want to interrupt sitting and you want to do it frequently and consistently.

Consider this: a study found the difference between those who were lean and those who were overweight came down to little movements during the day as small as bending over to pick up a piece of paper. Slim people did more of these little things. Another difference? Slimmer people moved more, being up and about for two hours more a day.

THINGS TO THINK ABOUT

- Small movements are beautiful ways to sculpt your body.
- Every step you take, every move you make causes positive changes to your body. Not moving is a BIG FAT mistake.
- Getting up every 20 minutes is a moving target.
- In terms of weight loss, this is truly a magical habit.
- Getting up to move is the best New Year's resolution ever, the best gift to your physical wellbeing and the best habit you can form for your weight and waistline.
- This is the simplest thing in the world.
- If you're going to form healthy habits, this is a keeper.

Understand old habits: launch new lifestyle

Easy enough to say—if you don't move, you don't lose.

That's all well and good but there can be reasons why habits of not moving have been created. And there are even more reasons for not moving enough to keep off the pounds.

Understanding these reasons can help you on the path to breaking the old habits and creating a new lifestyle.

Hereditary factors

"I inherited the fat gene," said our niece. She may have a point—at least when it comes to how much people move during the day and their weight. Research backs up the contention that there is a hereditary factor when it comes to weight and moving. The good news: with 21 days of effort we can overcome this possible obstacle. How? With 21 days of moving more and sitting less, our brains change to remind us to move more often.

This is the premise of researchers who, as noted earlier, found that some people move less and weigh more. Some people move more and are leaner. To study the issue, the researchers outfitted study participants in special movement measuring suits. Then the test subjects were fed specific meals consisting of more calories than needed. All were asked not to exercise.

At the end of a month, one group had gained an average of two and a half pounds, the other had maintained their original weight. Not only did the members of that group move more than they did originally, they moved even more unconsciously compensating for the additional calories they were given. The result was that they didn't gain weight.

Why would this be? Further research showed a heredity factor. Rats were injected (painlessly) with a chemical to make them move. Some rats, the obese ones, hardly reacted. Others, the lean ones, danced about. Researchers saw this as an indication that the tendency to move or not move was hard-wired into the brains of the rats.

Researchers concluded: how does all this relate to humans? What it means is that the brains of people with a tendency towards obesity don't respond to signals when their muscles or brains that tell them to move. And the more they sit, the fewer signals there are.

Don't despair. Don't start thinking your brain has hardwired you to be fat!

All is not lost because we can change our brains and the signaling mechanism. Dr. James Levine and his graduate student researchers involved in the above studies, encourage people to get up and walk every day. He notes the brain is adaptable and will change. Keep it up for three weeks. That's the amount of time needed for the brain to change.

By moving more, you'll be helping your brain remind your muscles to get up and move: it's a positive feed back loop.

Evolution and your weight

At this point in our evolution, we humans have an incredible amount of calories at our disposal. We don't have to expend calories hunting and gathering to obtain food as did our ancient ancestors. Food is easily available. We can decide to go out to lunch or walk into the kitchen to cook. On top of this, we have reduced the amount of moving needed to go through our days. The net result is too many calories and too little moving. It's a mismatch for our bodies. There are too many calories and not enough ways to expend them.

Of course, we'll accumulate weight. In addition, our bodies are built for survival. When we consume a bunch of calories, our bodies are designed to store calories as fat for times when there's famine. Research suggests we humans have an evolutionary tendency to conserve energy as a part of our survival mechanism. We need to conserve energy to survive. There is a fine line between this evolutionary need to conserve energy and the tipping point of conserving too much energy. The problem is that our body misreads the cultural norm of prolonged sitting as a situation in which the body is protecting itself. It's as if the body perceives sitting as it would an injury or some type of stress that is a threat.

There is a fine line between this evolutionary need to conserve energy and the tipping point of conserving too much energy.

This is not a matter of guilt trips and should-do-this/should-do-that. Think of this in an energy equation. Fat is storage of energy for future demands. But if you never actually place a demand, it just accumulates. The body doesn't understand. You just need to use a certain amount of calories over a certain amount of time or weight gain happens. The bodies handed down to us through the ages are pre-programmed to move for a critical period of time each day. Eons of days spent hunting and gathering food to survive pre-programmed muscles and metabolisms, setting them to engage our metabolism for a critical amount of time each day in the activities of standing and walking.

Consider this: standing up is a very difficult act. Moving is a very difficult act. Locomotion is a very difficult act. All require coordination of many systems. It requires a lot of energy. We are literally inhabiting a Neanderthal body built to move to survive.

The demands of our modern day life, are not enough to fire up the ancient inherited engines of our metabolisms.

Sit less and move more is not about a strenuous workout—it's about encouraging intermittent moving throughout the day

The good news: moving intermittently throughout the day can fill these needs. We weren't built to be long distance runners. We were built to sprint and chase animals, engaging our metabolisms in intermittent moving. This idea has entered into cardiovascular exercise with interval training. Interval training is built around the concept of sprinting for a short distance, resting and then sprinting again. This is not long distance running. Sit less and move more is not about a strenuous workout—it's about encouraging intermittent moving throughout the day.

I just don't move like I used to

"I just don't move like I used to."

Kevin says, *"I hear this all the time from people when I talk to them about the benefits of moving more."* His response to them: part of what I see is accumulation. It's the accumulation of not moving as much as you once did. Habits of not moving; injury and illness that discouraged movement in the are past lingering on, stress, depression and the feeling you can't make a move, are freezing into a pattern of life. It's a learning process. You learn that society discourages moving. You learn that you should sit still at school, at work, during social events. It's an act of conformity. Society is hell-bent on your sitting down and not moving. Don't rock the boat.

Remember being a kid? Running and moving all the time? We were processing our energy in a way that kept us thin and healthy. Is it time to put the kid back into your life?

Injury slows us down

Is an ankle sprain more than an ankle sprain? Does it potentially impact weight gain?

According to research, the answer is, yes. Research suggests "the effects of even a single ankle sprain, …potentially alters how well and often someone moves, for life."

The study showed that college students with chronic ankle instability, a condition caused by ankle sprains, in which the ankle easily gives way during movement, took 2,000 fewer steps a day than those with healthy ankles. Further research suggests the impact of an ankle sprain can last a lifetime. Research with mice showed that mice with injury move less throughout their lives…"

Is an ankle sprain more than an ankle sprain? Does it potentially impact weight gain?

How does this impact weight gain? Taking 2,000 fewer steps a day impacts not only calories expended but also found that activity is important for maintaining one's weight. Previous research has found that adding 2,000 steps to one's day helps one maintain weight. Taking 2,000 steps expends 100 calories. Not taking 2000 steps saves and stores those calories.

What about you? Have you been incapacitated by an ankle or other injury in the past? Staying still is a protective device to help you heal. You don't want to place weight on the ankle and complicate healing. You're protecting yourself from pain but, sustained over time, you're still using fewer steps. It's like energy renewal: when you move enough, walk enough you produce a sustainable supply of energy.

Maybe it's time to take a look at how you've recovered from an old injury. Have you gotten into the habit of not moving?

Time to take control

It's time to take control of your body. You become the master of your fate, the one who controls your weight. It's time to break free from the tyranny of sitting and liberate yourself from excessive weight.

What's your motivation? What does it for you?

Looking good in clothes? Fitting into your skinny clothes, the ones you bought or saved from a previous or hoped for weight level?

Feeling good about yourself? Or, as noted above, feeling good about looking at yourself in a mirror?

How about saving your life? How about having a good, active long life?

You need to tell yourself, I'm going to take the first step and the next one and the next one.

A focused effort will be more successful than an unfocused effort and it's how to make that focused effort that we're here to share with you.

Make up your mind that this is what you want to do. You need to tell yourself, I'm going to take the first step, and the next one and the next one. I'm going to build habits that will lead me to change my life.

The focused effort is: becoming aware of what you do now, how best to change it for a new you lifestyle and getting to your goal. From informal to formal we'll explore options that work for you.

And, here's the good part. You're in control. Want to make more progress? You can. Just move more, as Kevin says. But, like the game of tag, you're it. Only you can make it happen.

So let's do this. Let's get started.

Part two

LAUNCHING A NEW YOU

An intermittent moving you

5 Making a lifestyle decision

Let's get started launching a new you, one who is in control. You'll be creating a lifestyle of moving more and moving enough to lose weight and keep it gone.

First, take time to make the decision to launch a new lifestyle with new clear goals. Then, we'll be talking about what your body does all day and why it's important to your goals. Next, we'll look at what researchers have found to be a winning time frame for keeping pounds off.

We make decisions to stop smoking, change our diet or exercise. Yet, we don't even think about how much we sit, stand and move. All of these are connected. As studies show and as discussed above, the impact on us is profound.

By considering, and changing for the better such lifestyle habits, we change the very core of our well being.

Move more, sit less habits are lifestyle choices like those made about smoking, diet and exercise. By considering, and changing for the better such lifestyle habits, we change the very core of our well being. Whether you're consciously selecting it or not, the choice is there. Decide your fate:

Choose between the sitting lifestyle and the moving lifestyle.

As we discussed, there are any number of reasons for weight gain. But you CAN take control. Whatever may be challenging your weight, there are answers, practical and free things you can do to reach your weight loss goal.

More than likely, you've never even considered this: how much do you sit, stand and move throughout the day? It's time to become aware.

It's time to pay attention to what you and your body are doing. It's time to turn on your sit-stand-move mindfulness, and build an awareness of your sit-stand-move habits so you can make a success of your lifestyle. Make your lifestyle work for you.

What does your body spend its time doing?

What does your body do all day? Yes, the question is about your body, not you. This is an important question for those of us interested in losing some weight.

What lifestyle habit do you have at the moment? Do you sit all day? Do you sit all evening? Do you get up often to move around? Where do you spend your time sitting? On the way to work? At work? On the way home from work? At home in the evening? Every evening?

At issue is just one question: is your lifestyle making you fat?

At issue is just one question: is your lifestyle making you fat? Is your current lifestyle, what you're doing all day at work and all evening at home, at the heart of your weight problems?

Many obesity researchers now believe that the frequent, low level physical activities we do as we move through the day may have more to do with a healthy, weight controlled lifestyle than turning ourselves into gym rats.

For those who don't exercise (almost 80 percent of Americans), more than 90 percent of calories taken in each day, are consumed in light intensity physical activities such as walking to lunch, pacing while on the phone, cleaning the house, cooking, climbing stairs, standing while you talk to a friend, folding laundry.

It's time to start thinking about your current lifestyle so you can add more moving to your day.

Once again, what is it your body does all day? Sitting is probably what your body would say if it answered the question.

Your job is making you fat

Have you ever had the feeling your job is making you fat? If you feel that sitting all day at work contributes to your weight gain, you're right. Research backs you up and you're not alone.

Sitting for more than eight or nine hours a day at work translates into an increased risk for obesity (as well as diabetes and depression). The risk is less for people who move more often on the job.

If you feel that sitting all day at work contributes to your weight gain, you're right.

The workplace has changed over the years and with that change has come a weight-gain challenge. Since 1950, the number of jobs that require sitting has almost doubled. In the workplace of the 1980s, office workers spent 70 percent of their time sitting. Today it's 93 percent. According to one study, both men and women expend 100 calories less a day as they sit on the job today compared to 1970. Such changes in the workplace account for a significant portion of the average weight gain experienced by Americans over the years.

What can you do? What changes can be implemented by you to meet the challenge of avoiding weight gain in the workplace? You'll be reading about changes you can make in the following chapters.

You at home: the nightly collapse

Ready to spend your evening with your feet up in front of the television? Hunkered down in front of the computer? Sprawled in a chair or on the bed involved in Social Media on the cell phone? Streaming some video or playing an electronic game?

Welcome to the nightly collapse. This is a term Kevin created to describe what happens to many people, when they come home at the end of the day. Though they may be active at work or school all day, when they reach home, it's an entirely different story. It's ok to have a change of pace or a rest after a busy day, but you have to be aware of the timing of it. Yes, it's a well-deserved break but consider this: your body has its own schedule of metabolic needs. The nightly collapse can be a sabotage of your metabolism. You may not realize it but uninterrupted sitting is reversing the benefits of any activity you did during the day. And that includes all your carefully executed exercising. This has been shown in study after study.

Remember: it's not sitting that will put on the pounds. It's the continuity of it.

You can be on your feet all day long but your body doesn't understand what happens after work. It's what's happening now in the evening before bedtime, that your metabolism reacts to. It's the timing of it. To your body you're sitting for an extended period of time. This triggers that cascade of negative effects. This causes a kind of a metabolic chaos.

This is not to say you don't deserve to rest. It's all right to take a rest. It's just you want to rest smart. Resting smart takes several forms. You can take breaks from sitting and you can actively sit. (*See* Taking breaks from sitting, page 61 and Sitting smart, page 70). As you'll see, it's only takes a couple minutes to get your system and metabolism to rebound in the right direction.

Remember: it's not sitting that will put on the pounds. It's the continuity of it. You want to interrupt sitting and you want to do it frequently.

Are you an electronic couch potato?

You've heard of the couch potato? Meet the electronic couch potato, one who sits continuously while using an electronic device. And with the mobility of lap top computers, tablets and cell phones, this means that being a couch potato is no longer confined to the couch in the living room.

There is evidence that your computer use in the evening after work is making you fat. By extension, your tablet use and your smart phone use also contribute to your weight gain, It's not your electronic equipment that contributes to your weight gain but sitting while using it during your leisure time that does it. Children who use a tablet or cell phone for more than five hours a day had a 43 percent greater chance of becoming obese. In a study of young women, aged 20–24 who played computer games more than an hour a day it was shown that they were at risk for weight gain and obesity. Spending two hours or more a day chatting on line or emailing was also related to risk of weight gain for young women. Odds of obesity increased, for example, for those who used a computer eleven or more hours a week during their time off from work, compared with those who used computers for five or fewer hours per week.

Your television is making you fat

Ok, it's not your television itself that's making you fat. It's watching television while sitting for hours without a break. This is the origin of the couch potato.

Why would this be? Well, watching television is almost always done sitting. As with any seated activity, television watching translates into muscles that don't move resulting in lower metabolic activity and other weight gaining consequences. YIKES! your metabolism thinks, Inactivity! Store energy! Prepare for disaster!

Study after study shows television has more negative impact on the metabolic processes than other seated activities such as sewing, playing board games, reading, writing, or driving a car.

Ok, it's not your television itself that's making you fat. It's watching television while sitting for hours without a break.

Also as noted by one researcher: "television… is replacing everyday, non-sweaty movement as basic as standing and walking from room to room. The positive health effects of these seemingly negligible activities are underestimated. Modern technology has virtually engineered a lot of incidental, non-sweaty activity out of our lives."

This could be why studies show that the more hours spent in front of the tube translates into more likelihood for weight gain and obesity. But I like my television programs. Watching television is what I do to unwind at the end of a day.

We hear what you're saying and there are simple ideas to counteract the problem. Do something while watching television! It's really that simple. You'll be reading about what to do in Chapter 10. But right now it's important to realize what your body is doing during your off time.

Where do you fit in? How many hours of television time do you watch a day?

WHERE DO YOU FIT IN?

How many hours of seated television time do you usually do? What impact does it have on your weight and metabolism?

- If you sit and watch more than three continuous hours of television a day, you have a 90 percent risk of obesity.
- Those who exercised and watched three continuous hours of television typically were as fat as those who did not exercise.
- If your seated television viewing is in the four hour range, you are four times more likely to be overweight than people without this habit.
- Those who exercised and had four hours of seated television time were twice as likely to be overweight when compared to those who watched less than an hour of television per day and who did or did not exercise.
- If your seated television time reaches six hours a day you are four times more likely to be overweight than those who watched television or a VCR for an hour or less per week.

SEATED TELEVISION TIME AND YOUR METABOLISM

What impact does seated television time have on your metabolism?

One study found that each hour of television viewing increases the risk of metabolic syndrome. (In this study risk was defined as abnormal measures of three of five metabolic biomarkers)

- For women the risk was increased by 21 percent.
- For men the risk was increased by 26 percent.
- The odds for developing metabolic syndrome for women who sit more than four hours a day and do not exercise are 54 percent higher than for those women who sit less than one hour per day watching television and using the computer outside of work.
- For men, with more than four hours per day of seated screen time (television, computer, playing video games) outside of work, the odds for developing metabolic syndrome are even more dramatic:
- 94 percent higher odds (virtually double) of having metabolic syndrome.
- 88 percent higher odds of elevated waist circumference.
- 84 percent higher odds of low high-density lipoprotein cholesterol (HDL-C).
- 55 percent higher odds of high blood pressure.
- 32 percent higher odds of elevated glucose.

In addition to weight gain, all of these are contributing factors to heart attack, stroke, diabetes, Alzheimer's disease and early death.

In children, seated television watching has been shown to impact mental processes and behavior.

Binge watching is making you fat

Can't resist whiling away the weekend or evening binge watching? What could be better than seeing an entire season of your favorite show all at once? No commercials means there's no natural break time to visit the kitchen or bathroom. Sitting for hours—it's easy when you're entertained. Binge watching is like seated television hours on steroids.

You've seen the numbers above for television watching. The same statistics hold true for binge watching.

It's decision time.

6 The new, determined you

Moving more and sitting less throughout your day is the key to your success. It's about your expenditure of energy.

If you spend it wisely, you're going to reap untold benefits. You'll help reduce your risk for weight gain and metabolic dysfunction. You can lose weight and avoid some common health challenges. Remember, this is how you're going to lose weight; this is how you're going to lose waistline inches, this is how you're going to feel healthy all day long. This is how you can regain the you that is energetic and aligned for health. Keep your goal in mind.

What you do as you move through your day is important. Why? As noted previously, more than 90 percent of calories we use during the day are used doing the simple things we normally do as we move through the day. It's what you do the most. It's the walking. It's going up and down stairs. It's bending over to pick up a stray piece of paper on the floor. It's cooking and cleaning and doing laundry. It's picking up the newspaper and taking out the trash. It's all the little things that are going to make you a success.

...more than 90 percent of calories we use during the day are used doing the simple things we normally do as we move through the day.

It is the intermittent moving between bouts of sitting that's going to make you happy and successful because it's going to eat up more calories as well as reset your metabolism and appetite. After awhile you're not going to think about it; you'll just get up and move.

Kevin's Story

My pants fell off in the driveway long after I quit thinking about making an effort to move. Moving more had become a natural habit. It makes me happy now because I've lost weight. It makes me happy because this is an achievable goal. I've added more movement to my life. I go to the gym. I bounce on the mini-tramp. I walk. I just enjoy the sense that I am in control. It's like spending habits. You want money in the bank. You make a budget and start accumulating it. With moving more, you go about accumulating the benefits of your good habits.

It's the happiness habit. It's knowing every step you take is moving you toward your goal, your success your feeling of control. This is what you need to focus on. It's the background noise of more movement.

Move more, sit less to improve

What is the new lifestyle that will help you control your weight? It's shifting time spent sitting to time spent up and about. It's one where increasing moving time and lessening sitting time leads you to weight loss and a smaller waistline. It's the intermittent moving lifestyle. It's timing and adjusting your sitting, standing and moving activities to optimize your metabolism, calorie expenditure and appetite control.

Kevin's Story

Once again: when I talk to people about my weight loss experience and the research, what I try to emphasize is this: you can do everything right. You can eat the best food. You can exercise. But if you're not moving enough throughout the day, it can go for naught. Your body does not understand long periods of not moving. We were built to move. That's the prime directive.

I like to emphasize and re-emphasize this point. Why? Because it's something no one's ever told you in your efforts at weight loss. This is not an exercise program. This is a lifestyle.

Why did I start moving more? Barbara kept telling me what she was discovering as she dug into the research for a new book about what happens as we sit too much. All the research pointed in the same direction. Small continual movements throughout the day were key to good health. The impact of many small movements through out the day ranges far and wide from decreased risks for health problems both physical and mental from diabetes, stroke, heart disease, Alzheimer's, depression and more—including obesity.

Kevin is not alone. Once people find out what's going on, they get up and moving too. One researcher studied sitting and what she found got her moving. She lost 40 pounds. (What her research found: the more people sit, the shorter their life expectancies.) A writer who looked into the issue of sitting, got moving and lost 15 pounds. The artist, who started standing for part of the day to paint, lost 23 pounds. More about them later.

It's about timing. It's basically about how much you move and when you move.

The simple act of getting up and moving for two minutes is easy. The hard part is keeping yourself motivated and consistent to change your metabolism.

The simple part is the technique. The hard part is keeping it consistent, staying on track. The simple act of getting up and moving for two minutes is easy. Yes, you can find time in your day to move more. The hard part is keeping yourself motivated and consistent to change your metabolism. Bar none, that is the hardest part. But, we're here to help you with tips and ideas and motivation. The best part—this is free. There is no cost to it.

Absolutely no cost whatsoever. It's you and your effort, taking control and creating the you who you want to be.

A LIFESTYLE INTERVENTION

A lifestyle intervention to sit less and move more was the suggestion of Australian researchers.

Following a study with participants who were diabetic and overweight, they found that shifting time from a prolonged sedentary lifestyle to a non-prolonged sedentary or light-intensity activity lifestyle significantly improved both waistline and body mass index.

7 The intermittent moving lifestyle

With the intermittent moving lifestyle, you're still sitting, you're still standing, you're still moving just as you do every day. You're just changing how often you do each.

You sit but you stand more and, especially, move more. By adjusting the amounts of how much time you spend sitting, standing and moving, you burn more calories, as well as adjust a slowed metabolism and your appetite control.

Sure, we all realize if we move more, more calories are expended. Are you a motivated counter of the calories you consume? Do you also keep track when you expend those calories? (More on this later.)

Are you a motivated counter of the calories you consume?

Where does metabolism come in to our sitting, standing and moving habits? Well, automatic reflexes kick in as we sit, stand or move. And, when we don't move often enough, these reflex actions, important to our metabolisms, are thrown off. Disrupted are our fat vacuums, blood sugar levels, natural appetite controls, blood pressure and more. All these impact our weight and waistlines and our health.

There are three modes of activity for your body: sit, stand, move. It's all about timing. It's about the amount of time you're spending in each mode. If we sit and don't move in a certain amount of time, unwanted things happen.

The benefits of moving more and sitting less: weight control

Does it seem that some people you know just never seem to gain weight? There may be a reason.

As mentioned earlier, they move more and sit less. At least that's what one study found. Why would this be? A further study showed that people appear to be born with a propensity to be either fidgety or listless. It seems there is a natural, genetic tendency to move more or less during the day.

Leaner participants moved two and a quarter hours more and sat two and a quarter hours less than the heavier participants.

Heavier people sit more and move less during the day. Lean people move more and sit less during the day. What was amount of time and activity that made a difference between those who were lean and those who were heavy? Two hours and fifteen minutes. Heavier study participants sat two and a quarter hours more and so moved two and a quarter hours less each day than the leaner participants.

Leaner participants moved two and a quarter hours more and sat two and a quarter hours less than the heavier participants.

Researchers who conducted the study and found these results also noted: the extra motion by lean people is enough to burn about 350 extra calories a day, which could add up to 10 to 30 pounds a year.

There's more: leaner people engaged in more minor movements like picking up a scrap of paper from the floor, according to the study by researcher Dr. James A. Levine of the Mayo Clinic.

It's about timing

It's about timing when it comes to the move more, sit less prescription. We're all familiar with the phrase minimum daily requirements when they are referring to vitamins. But our bodies too, have minimum daily requirements—for moving.

And, yes exercise is important and deserves its own category but exercise is no replacement for what you do all day. Exercise is no replacement for the little, the medium and the larger sized bits of moving.

The biggest thing Kevin found in his weight loss quest? It's about time and timing. You can stand all you want. You can move all you want. But if you go for long periods of not moving, your system simply shuts down. Start moving. Start losing.

We'll guide you through ideas to add movement to your day and evening and help you to overcome impediments to moving.

Moving to your body's own natural rhythms

How to reach your goal of weight loss by moving more and sitting less? It's about matching what you do throughout your day and how your body works. It's about your body's own natural rhythms. Meet your body's needs to move and you'll unlock the path to weight loss and control.

Central to the timing that is crucial to your weight are three things. First is what we call intermittent moving. This is simply taking breaks from sitting. The result is that you get up and move regularly throughout the day. Think of this as bite-sized bits: a little sitting here, a little moving there all, accomplished by taking breaks from sitting throughout your day and evening.

Meet your body's needs to move and you'll unlock the path to weight loss and control.

Next is taking a little walk after meals. A little walk could simply be circuits around your living room. A 10 to 15 minute walk helps re-set your blood sugar demand, following a meal. (High blood-sugar levels increase risk for diabetes, a risk especially important to those with weight concerns as noted earlier. In addition, research has found that walking helps speed up the time it takes food to move from the stomach into the small intestines. This may help you feel full after eating.

Finally and maybe most important, is moving enough during the day. For most people it's a matter of adding steps to those they already take throughout the day. How can you add steps to your busy day? First, you'll want to count the steps you take. It's motivational when you see those steps add up. It's easy to do with today's technology. Use a pedometer, your cell phone app or wearable technology such as a FitBit or VivoFit. As you'll read below, taking breaks from sitting and a little walk after meals will practically make your goal of increasing your steps per day to over 10,000. Soon you'll be impacting your weight and waistline.

8 Harnessing the move more, sit less lifestyle

Harnessing the intermittent moving lifestyle is a matter of thinking about and changing how much time you spend sitting, standing and moving about.

You don't need a gym, a set of barbells or a spandex outfit. There's only one requirement. You and your determination to reboot your metabolism and appetite control.

Every time you stand up, you reboot your body. You cause your metabolism to change. You signal your appetite control. You break up the pattern detrimental to your weight that forms from sitting too long.

> *Every time you stand up, you reboot your body. You cause your metabolism to change.*

It's conditioning. You are conditioning how your metabolism acts. When you start, you're interrupting a metabolic pattern. If you interrupt it consistently and do it long enough, your body starts to repair this metabolic pattern gone awry. If you make it a lifetime habit, your body enters a state of wellness where your metabolism is functioning properly. You're maintaining your weight. You're maintaining your waistline. You have more energy.

It's simple. It's free.

Do you want to change your metabolism? Everyone says, yes, to that question. You want to interrupt sitting and you want to do it frequently, frequently enough so that your metabolism resets.

Sitting is not the problem. It's not moving that's the problem.

Focus on your goal to gain control

As you make decisions about moving more throughout your day, be mindful of what you are gaining. By consciously considering what you spend your time doing, you are gaining control of what you may have considered an out-of-control situation, your weight. Every footstep and every break in sitting moves you closer to your goal. Interrupt your sitting and interrupt it often.

Subtle factors come into play. If you sprain your ankle, you're going to sit more. Or if you've sprained your ankle in the past, maybe you've gotten accustomed to sitting more. Or, maybe you've got a knee problem where moving is a problem. Then there's social pressure. If you're the only person standing up in a room of seated people, you'll want to sit. Resist. Remember your goals. you are simply standing, not breaking any rules.

One simple act, one simple behavior change could change your waistline, your weight, your cognitive abilities, your cholesterol levels, your blood sugar levels. It's the intermittent lifestyle. It's a habit for a better outcome for you and your body.

One simple act, one simple behavior change could change your waistline, your weight, your cognitive abilities, your cholesterol levels, your blood sugar levels.

It's the simplest thing in the world to do: stand up and move. It's the hardest thing in the world to do and keep doing. It's a world built around not moving: energy saving, easy living. It's what everyone else is doing, It's a world is constructed around the conformity of not moving.

The goal: lose weight, lose waistline, live smarter, live better, live longer.

What's it going to take to get you moving?

Focus, evaluate your results and re-focus

As you develop your moving more and sitting less lifestyle, focus on how well it's working. Is it convenient, fitting easily into your day? Do you find yourself really moving more and sitting less? And, are you getting results? If not, why not?

It may be time to re-focus your efforts. Look over the intermittent moving techniques and see if another one might work better for you. If it's a matter of motivating yourself, *see* Troubleshooting, page 112.

Make life less convenient or "don't put your Beermeister next to your recliner."

This piece of life advice was passed on by one of Kevin's health-challenged reflexology clients. While many of us choose not to live with a beer-dispensing machine in the living room, the overall message is one to take to heart when choosing to move more and sit less.

Make life less convenient.

Labor saving isn't saving us.

Take an attitude that all the labor saving devices and technology we now have are working against us. Labor saving isn't saving us. It's a push button society with saving steps and easy chairs. There's a steady drip, drip, drip of inactivity. But that's not the root cause. The root cause is not technology. The root cause has a lot to do with how much you're NOT moving.

The banker at our local bank comes to mind. Her office cubicle is set up very efficiently with everything at her fingertips. From her chair she can easily reach a phone, printer, a Fax machine and a copy machine. No need to venture out of her cubicle. Over the years I've seen the pounds accumulate. I am sure she is aware of it, too.

If something's a block away, do you walk or take the car? If you want to go from the first floor to the second floor, do you take the elevator instead of the stairs? We've been conditioned. There's a whole school of thought devoted to the value of taking the stairs. End labor saving. Just because it's easier doesn't mean it's good for you. Just because you could, doesn't mean you should get on that elevator.

Building awareness, being mindful

By the act of being aware, you're on the path to changing how things work. You will burn more calories. You will eliminate fat in your blood more efficiently. You will move blood sugar in you blood more effectively. You will signal your body's natural appetite control to be more accurate.

Overall, your metabolism will be better, implementing a whole host of health improvements. You will become aware that your body is more than just a platform for what your mind is doing.

By the act of being aware, you're on the path to changing how things work.

How often have you sat for long periods of time, not even conscious of it? Is it possible you've sat for hours at times and not really been aware? We have all been so absorbed in our tasks that we lose track of time. We have all worked to meet that deadline. We're all guilty of this. But it's time for a new lifestyle, one where you're mindful of what you're doing and doing it with your goal in mind.

Helping yourself lose weight

What happens when you become more aware of what you do?

You can literally change your life. You can change the way you look. You can change the way you feel. You can even change the way you think about things.

And, there can also be those valuable weight loss ramifications.

One study found that being mindful in itself helped weight loss. One group of study participants lost two pounds more in a month than those in the other group. The difference? Those in the one group were made aware that their daily routine was the same as a beneficial exercise session. The study was conducted with hotel maids as subjects.

One group of hotel maids was informed and then reminded that the jobs they did every day met the Surgeon General's suggested exercise recommendations. They were also alerted to the number of calories expended as they vacuumed and scrubbed their way through the day.

Members of this group lost an average of two pounds as well as improved their blood pressure by ten points. Their body fat and waist to hip measurements also improved when compared to the maids in the group who were not told their work was beneficial exercise.

Imagine the effort it takes to lose two pounds. Now imagine losing weight merely by being aware that your move more, sit less effort is a beneficial exercise for your body.

Imagine every step you take feeding your metabolism and appetite control what they need to work better!

By becoming aware and giving yourself credit for your sit less and move more habits, you'll move forward with your weight loss goals

The lesson to be learned: thinking about what you do makes a difference to your body. This is mindfulness.

By becoming aware and giving yourself credit for your sit less and move more habits, you'll move forward with your weight loss goals.

Action ideas

Start your awareness and mindfulness campaign. By observing the blocks of time you spend sitting, standing and moving, you start to get a picture of your current lifestyle.

Is it your habit to sit for long periods of time? Talk, text or check social media on the cell phone? Watch television? Binge watch Netflix?

There are ways to become more aware of how long you've sat. What would work for you? Is it a timer, set to time your sitting?

Post-it notes serving as reminders, placed where you can see them as you sit? Keeping tabs on the clock on the wall? Using your smart phone to time your sitting?

Are you a calorie counter?

Some work to lose weight by counting the number of calories in what they eat. If you are included in this group, did you ever think to factor your actual calorie calculations as calories expended?

If you're sitting and not moving, you're not spending the calories you could. It's time to think about moving and spending those calories.

Yes, getting up and moving is worth calories. For example, sitting for an hour expends 75 calories. Moving for an hour expends 150 calories. As you read through the following techniques, you'll find calorie spending information is provided for many of them.

Part three

MOVE MORE, SIT LESS TECHNIQUES

9 Focusing your efforts

Feel free to move more and sit less as you please. But if you're interested in focusing your efforts, you'll be more effective. Why not use techniques that have been found to have a value and have been tested by research?

Whether you're considering your metabolism, counting calories, or telling yourself how your appetite control is improving, we want you to be aware that you're doing good for yourself.

Essentially, we can show you not only ideas for getting up and moving but also what's in it for you—what you gain and what you lose. And these techniques are not just happy thoughts but research-tested benefits for your efforts.

We'll be showing you how to focus your efforts as you:
• Sit less, move more.
• Take breaks from sitting.
• Sit smart.
• Do something while watching television.
• Taking steps to take steps.
• House cleaning (really, it has a value beyond neatening up).
• Have some fun: stand and direct or dance to the music, stand and cheer your sports team, play some active video gaming.

You can try any of the techniques we mention or you can invent your own. Allow yourself to change your strategy over time. Again, if motivation is your stumbling block, check out the Troubleshooting section on page 112.

Do you talk yourself out of moving? If you need strategies

to implement an intermittent moving lifestyle, *see* the Troubleshooting section on page 112. Don't be afraid to change and try something new. This is a process.

Let's get ready to un-sit your lifestyle. To start, we present stories of people who have succeeded and how they did it. Next, we'll go on to talk more about the techniques you can use. To add to your motivation, we'll explain why they work.

See yourself succeeding: stories of those who have

What would your day be like if you moved more and sat less? Can you imagine it? Can you see it?

It's easy to say: move more and sit less the right amount of time and positive things will happen for your metabolism and weight-control. The reality is different. It's about forming a healthy habit. It's about fitting the time of moving more and sitting less into your lifestyle. What's important is what works for you.

What would your day be like if you moved more and sat less? Can you imagine it? Can you see it?

You'll get to customize this to your lifestyle so you are successful. Remember to be kind to yourself. Realize who you are and what you do. Work with that.

As you read the following stories of success, note how each individual tailored a program to fit his or her day. Think about what you do during your day. Gather more ideas for your personal lifestyle in order to be this better you.

Kevin

Kevin replaced his office desk with a standing desk. For evening entertainment he created a standing station from a plant stand to hold his iPad. Underfoot he placed a textured reflexology mat. He could then move in place rather than stay still. He walked for 30 minutes every day. (He had walked for years and experienced weight loss only after he un-sat his life.) He lost 40 pounds and eight inches off his waistline in six months.

Kevin's gone on to other strategies. One is taking 10,000 or more steps a day. He uses an Apple Watch to count steps. Yes, he can be a real techno nerd! Some of his steps are taken walking in place on reflexology mats. He also bounce-steps in place on a mini trampoline for 15 minutes after each meal. His weight and waistline loss continue to be under control and growing smaller.

Dr. Alpa Patel and the American Cancer Society

Researcher Dr. Alpa Patel of the American Cancer Society, studied the impact of sitting on longevity. (The findings: women who sat more than six hours a day during their time off, had a 33 percent higher risk of early death from cardiovascular disease than women who only sat three hours. The figure was 18 percent for men.)

Impressed by the results Dr. Patel, embarked on her own move more and sit less program. Dr. Patel did just three things.
1. She parked her car away from her building at work.
2. She took stairs instead of the elevator whenever she could, and
3. She moved every hour for a few minutes. These are not radical or difficult activities. In addition, she tried active sitting (sitting on an exercise ball at the office to engage her postural muscles and burn more calories). She began to stand during conference calls. She used a printer in another office that gave her a reason to get up and walk a bit. She began to walk over to a colleague's office instead of emailing them. She took a brisk 20-minute walk at lunch, she began adding longer walks before or after work. She lost 40 pounds in six months. None of this required buying gym clothes, gym membership or gym equipment. None of this required gym time.

Edward does it with art

Professional artist Edward now paints with his easel on a sit-stand device. Instead of sitting all the time as he paints, he now stands to paint sometimes and he sits and paints sometimes. He's lost 23 pounds in three months.

Actor John Goodman takes steps

Making sure to take 10,000 to 12,000 steps a day helped actor John Goodman lose 100 pounds over two years. The actor also followed a Mediterranean diet and exercised six days a week.

Claudia, the stay-at-home mom

One stay-at-home mom added steps to her life. Whenever she went to the grocery store, she planned to walk every aisle even if the items she needed were not on those shelves. She also made extra trips to and from her laundry room while doing the family laundry. She folded and put away the laundry by category and location. Different categories and different locations were different trips. This may not seem like an efficient system but it efficiently helped her efficiently lose four and a half pounds in the first month. Using a Fitbit, she calculated she was taking up to 15,000 steps a day.

Each of these people discovered their own intermittent moving lifestyle routines that worked to create their weight loss. They found that critical tipping point that matched their lifestyles to their bodies' needs to move.

10 Managing your sitting time

Sit less, lose more! Why sit less? It's a cornerstone of weight gain and weight loss: by expending more calories you are signaling your metabolism and appetite control systems to help you.

More calories are expended by moving than by sitting. But it's not just about using more calories as you move. It's about signaling your body. It's about triggering the right signals to get your body to quit eating, its appetite control.

> *It's about triggering the right signals to get your body to quit eating, its appetite control.*

It's about accurately gauging your need for fuel. It can be a bottomless pit. You just eat and eat and eat when you don't have the right signal going on. What's going to happen when you eat a surplus of calories that don't match your movement? You're going to store those calories as fat.

Again, research shows those who sit the most have the poorest indicators for metabolic health connected to weight. Prolonged sitting has powerful metabolic consequences. Prolonged sitting disrupts metabolic processes that break down fats and sugars in the blood. How to change this?

One strategy is to keep track of how much you're sitting each day. A smart phone app can help you keep track. Knowing the size of the problem is part of solving the problem. Another solution that many people like is the simple one of keeping track of how often one takes breaks from sitting and how much one moves. Timing breaks can be achieved using an egg timer or a similar device or your cell phone. How much one moves can be a matter of counting steps using a pedometer, a smart phone or a FitBit or some other wearable technology that has a step counter.

Read on for more about sitting less, timing and your weight loss goals.

Take breaks from sitting

Taking breaks from sitting is not hard to do. Stand up. Leave your chair. Walk.

What's important is what it does for your body. It creates a pattern of intermittent moving crucial to keeping your metabolism working at its best.

Taking breaks from sitting is the simplest and easiest way to move more and sit less.

Taking breaks from sitting is the simplest and easiest way to move more and sit less. And the good news for weight loss seekers is that more calories are used up and you reset your metabolism.

Taking breaks is so important, please forgive us as we go into more detail again! Read on to discover:
• Benefits of taking breaks from sitting.
• Taking breaks from sitting: how long and how often.
• What to do when taking a break? Standing vs. walking.
• Breaks with a purpose.
• Commercial stepping.

For tips about taking breaks on the job, *see* chapter 12, pages 87–99.

If you have physical limitations that make standing up and sitting down difficult, consider Active Sitting, page 70.

Benefits of taking breaks from sitting

What can taking breaks from sitting do for you and your quest to improve your weight?

MUSCULOSKELETAL BENEFITS

Among benefits is the lessening of musculoskeletal discomfort. Author Barbara changed office chairs several times hoping to find a better sitting platform to lessen neck pain. Once she started taking breaks from sitting every 15 minutes, neck pain was no longer a problem. Why would this be? Standing places the skeleton in a more natural position, creating less stress on the spine, than sitting in a chair. Barbara is free of the chronic neck pain that she had endured for years.

First, a few stories. Kevin's client was a businesswoman who described her work process as lock and load. She stayed in her home office chair for four hour bouts of non-stop sitting and concentrated on work. She was puzzled why weight continued to be a problem considering she got up faithfully at five a.m. multiple times a week to attend a spin class.

For another of Kevin's clients, a busy lawyer, four non-stop hours was a light day at work. She frequently sat for longer. It never occurred to her to link her hours of sitting to her weight concerns.

What's the common element here?

Uninterrupted sitting without moving is detrimental to metabolic functions related to weight. Good cholesterol, triglycerides, blood pressure and blood glucose levels as well as waistline size are all connected to this. In summary in case this is not branded on your brain now:
• Taking breaks from sitting re-sets metabolic mechanisms related to your weight gain.
• The more breaks taken from sitting throughout the day, the more improvement you will see in those metabolic indicators connected to obesity.

- The number of small breaks from sitting are more important
  to the size of one's waistline than exercise. Those who take
  the most breaks throughout the day had a smaller waistline
  by one and a half inches compared to those who take the least
  number of breaks. (An inch and a half is the clothing industry's
  marker between one size of clothing and the next smaller size
  of clothing.)
- Taking breaks from sitting causes more calories
  to be used up than sitting quietly.

Blood flow to the brain is another thing improved
when breaks are taken from sitting. A two-minute
break from sitting keeps the flow of blood to the
brain constant, ensuring appropriate nutrients
and oxygen reach the brain. This could explain
other research results showing children learn and
behave better when they take breaks from sitting.
Creativity is shown to be increased when adults take breaks
during their workday.

The number of small breaks from sitting are more important to the size of one's waistline than exercise.

A break in sitting every 30 minutes is associated with a decreased
risk for death. Those who took breaks, compared to those
who sat throughout the day without the breaks had improved
longevity.

Taking breaks from sitting: how long and how often
Taking breaks from sitting is an important part of reaching your
goals. It's an opportunity to reset your metabolism, increase
calorie expenditure and create a smaller waistline. How long and
how often should breaks be in order to get you to your goals? It
will be different for every person. But we just can't say it enough.

Taking breaks in sitting activates and normalizes the body's
metabolism thrown into disarray by sitting:
- Within 90 seconds of standing, the muscular and cellular
  systems that process three of the five parts of metabolism
  important to weight (blood sugar, triglycerides, and cholesterol)
  are activated.

- A two-minute break from sitting every 20 minutes resets important components of metabolism—your blood pressure and your blood sugar metabolism.
- A break in sitting every 30 minutes improves indicators of obesity: these include the Body Mass Index (a weight-to-height ratio used as an indicator of obesity and underweight), waist circumference and fat percentage. (Metabolism slows by 90 percent after 30 minutes of sitting.)
- A five-minute break from sitting every hour helps create feelings of greater happiness, and less fatigue and less craving for food.
- If you have been sitting one hour, you have been sitting too long. Your cellular processes, important to metabolism, are already slowing down.

If you have been sitting one hour, you have been sitting too long. Your cellular processes, important to metabolism, are already slowing down.

Taking breaks from sitting every 30-minutes provides an opportunity to use up more calories. Over an eight-hour work day:

- A one minute break results in the expenditure of an additional 24 calories.
- A two-minute break results in 59 extra calories expended.
- A five- minute break results in an 132 additional calories expended.

Thus a five-minute break taken every hour for eight hours for five days is equal to the calories in a big pile of French fries.

Not much you might think? Remember: one study found sitting jobs resulted in the lessened expenditure of 100 calories a day. This is enough to account for a significant portion of the weight gain experienced by women and men in the U.S. over the past fifty years.

What do you do when taking a break? Standing vs. walking

What do you do when taking a break? It makes a difference. The best option: walking around.

MAGIC 20-MINUTE BREAKS

Is 20 minutes a magic number for taking breaks from sitting?

Research into longevity provides a clue. Engage in physical activity every 20 minutes and you'll live healthier and longer. Dan Buettner, author of *The Blue Zones Solution: Eating and Living Like the World's Healthiest People*, found cultures around the world whose residents live the healthiest and longest are "nudged into physical activity (such as house work, yard work, kitchen work (in a kitchen) with no mechanized appliances) every 20 minutes. This type of activity not only burned 500 to 1,000 calories a day; it also kept their metabolisms humming at a high rate."

As noted earlier, 90 seconds of standing activates several measures of metabolism. Other researchers have found walking is an even better way to re-set metabolism. Why would this be? Walking burns three times the calories of sitting. Standing expends almost the same number of calories as sitting. Research showed that those who stood up while taking a break from sitting expended only two or three calories more in 15 minutes than they did while they were seated for 15 minutes. When walking for 15 minutes, however, they expended 32 calories more than they did while seated. They used up 32 calories for every 15 minutes that they walked. In an hour of strolling, this is equal to about 130 more calories that are used when just sitting. (It may sound small but remember we are looking at cumulative results, and triggering better health.)

Other things happen as well when as we walk. Its not just things that have to do with metabolism.

Muscles as they move us, improve us. By taking up glucose from the blood as well as activating the enzymes that break down blood fats (triglycerides), movement causes levels of the good cholesterol to rise, too. Lower levels of that enzyme are linked to a myriad of lifestyle conditions such as obesity, atherosclerosis, Alzheimer's disease, metabolic syndrome, and a condition associated with diabetes, insulin resistance.

... next time you take a break from sitting, take full advantage of your time. Don't just stand there. Move!

The up-shot: next time you take a break from sitting, take full advantage of your time. Don't just stand there. Move! Move for two minutes or more.

Breaks with a purpose

Having a purpose, having something to do during your time up and about, might give you extra incentive to get up and get moving.

- One woman had a practical and unique plan to get up and get moving: she drinks a glass of water every hour. Getting out of her chair to get the glass of water or the resulting trip to the bathroom gets her up and gets her moving. Her FitBit now less frequently prompts her to take a break from sitting.
- Did you make a mess in the area surrounding your favorite easy chair? Neaten up, carry the glasses and dishes to the kitchen, and take the newspapers to your recycling bin. Take those steps.
- Perform a short housecleaning detail such as emptying the dishwasher or moving the wet laundry to the dryer.
- Water plants.
- Play with your pets.
- Play with your children.

YOUR OWN COMMERCIAL TIME

Binge watching? Create your own commercial time

- Use the pause button on your remote.
- Set a timer to remind yourself to interrupt your sitting, Get up and move!

Commercial stepping—it's not what you think!
Need a reminder to get up and take breaks while watching
television? Commercial stepping may be for you.

What's commercial stepping? It's standing up and taking steps
while commercials are playing on your television. Do you really
need to see that advertising? Step in place or walk around the
room. Just get up and get moving. You won't miss anything
important on the tube.

The timing of commercials is just right to have a healthy
impact—they will come on about every 20 minutes. They
last at least 90 seconds—just the time needed to re-set your
metabolism. And there's the benefit of not watching something
designed to make you buy something.

In addition, there's the benefit of using calories. When you stand
up and walk in place during those pesky commercial breaks, an
hour of television viewing can add up 148 calories used up. This
is 67 calories more than the 81 calories you burn
while just sitting in your easy chair. Sixty-seven
calories is equal to walking a quarter of a mile.

*Taking breaks from
sitting has benefits
beyond weight gain.*

If you're counting steps (*see* Taking steps,page 75),
an added bonus is the 2,000 steps taken in an hour.

One study found an hour of television watching includes 16 to
24 minutes of commercials. Stepping in place during one hour
of commercials resulted in an average of about 25 minutes of
physical activity.

Further benefits of taking breaks from sitting
Taking breaks from sitting has benefits beyond weight gain.
Consider the following findings.

Cancer prevention
Taking frequent breaks in sitting for as little as one minute
can lower the biomarkers associated with risk for cancer (waist

circumference, insulin resistance and inflammation)—all indicators of cancer risk common to many physical activity-cancer studies.

Blood pressure, insulin/glucose, metabolism/cardiovascular risk

Taking a two-minute break in sitting every 20 minutes re-sets the body's mechanisms that you have put under stress by sitting. Lessened are risks for diabetes, cancer, cardiovascular disease, and metabolic syndrome.

Blood pressure Two-minute breaks in sitting every 20 minutes lowered both systolic and diastolic blood pressure by three points.

Insulin/glucose metabolism/lessened cardiovascular risk Two-minute breaks every 20 minutes over a five-hour period following a meal resulted in lower glucose and insulin levels compared to just sitting for five hours after a meal.

A two–three-minute break every 20 or 30 minutes helps relieve the musculoskeletal stress on the hips and lower back.

Musculoskeletal stress

A two–three-minute break every 20 or 30 minutes helps relieve the musculoskeletal stress on the hips and lower back created by sitting too long. Sitting impacts the role that your hips and lower back play in providing a stable base for walking. Over time as you age, your ability to move and your risk of possible injury when moving can increase.

Intermittent moving can lessen the risk of work related injuries and injuries from sports. And all of this can lead to a diminished ability to walk in later life.

In addition, intermittent movement can affect the chance of developing a potbelly and a big butt.

Musculoskeletal discomfort on the job (think sore stiff neck and aching back)

Breaks of any length of time can help a stiff neck or aching back. Consider stretching and simply walking away from your workstation for a moment.

Could you manage a micro-break of 30 seconds every 20 minutes? That would be four breaks an hour for 120 seconds. That would be the equivalent of a two-minute break. What about a five-minute break every hour (aside from regular mid-morning, mid-afternoon and lunch breaks?) Could you manage that? Could you manage living well and living longer?

Author Barbara continued searching for the best office chair to stave off neck pain. Taking breaks in prolonged sitting research ended her search. It wasn't a better chair she needed, it was regular breaks from sitting in the chair!

Learning for children, performance for adults

Moving about every 20 minutes improves student behavior and enhances the learning experience for children. It improves brain development, increases nerve connections, and solidifies learning skills. The same is true for adult learning performance.

According to brain researcher Eric Jensen: movement improves brain development, increases nerve connections, and solidifies learning... These energizers (moving frequently) wake up learners, increase their energy levels, improve their information storage and retrieval and helps them feel good. A very short break or energizer increases brain arousal but longer breaks allow the learner to be brain aroused and come back from a break with a more sustainable level of energy.

Do something while you're watching television or binge watching

Do something while you're watching television. Don't just sit there: be active while watching television or streaming programming.

Position fitness equipment in the room. Anything that will get you up and moving while watching is good: you can use a yoga mat, a mini-trampoline, an exercycle, or a rowing or machine. For example, Harvard researcher Dr. Frank Hu has a treadmill in front of the television so he can get some exercise while watching the news.

Go barefoot! A jute welcome mat, a bath mat or any textured surface underfoot creates more benefit than just standing.

Increase your standing and moving time by creating a standing platform to hold a book, iPad, tablet, laptop or other entertainment device. Create a standing station from a fern stand or any other tall object with a flat top. A music stand left over from your days as a student in the school band is an inexpensive and an adjustable platform. Go barefoot! A jute welcome mat, a bath mat or any textured surface underfoot creates more benefit than just standing. Sway in place or move just a bit when you stand up.

Sit smart, be active while sitting. Read on!

Sitting smart: active sitting

Get ready to sit smart, using more calories than normal quiet sitting. Your metabolism will thank you and improve as well.

Yes, there can be more to sitting than just sitting quietly. It turns out what you do while sitting is important, too. Sit smart, sit with a purpose, making every moment count.

Sitting smart includes considering your chair, your environment for time spent sitting, as well as active sitting techniques.

There are a variety of active sitting techniques that are simple yet provide benefits. Even more, you're stacking activities, doing something that will improve both your body and mind. Rocking, for example, causes more blood to be sent to the heart and brain. Improved are your blood pressure, your brainpower and your mood. Rocking chairs aren't just for babies and grandmothers.

Active sitting: rocking in a rocking chair
As long as you're sitting there, you might as well be getting some benefit out of it: rocking in a rocking chair eats up twice the calories as sitting quietly (150 per hour versus 75) and more.

While most of us call it a rocking chair others have a different take. Some researchers call it a medical device or a therapy. By any name, rocking creates improvements in physical and mental well-being.

Yes, the rocking chair in your living room can become your mini gym. It is a mild form of exercise for the elderly or for those who have difficulties walking or individuals coping with knee problems.

Why would this be?

Rocking with your toes pointed mimics the same activity that takes place as we stand or walk:
• As the muscles of the calves contract and relax, the veins located within them compress and decompress Thus blood is pumped from the extremities and returned to the brain and heart.
• The rocking motion stimulates the vestibular apparatus of the inner ears which is tied to maintaining balance when walking. How important is this? Lack of balance is the number one contributor to injuries from falls among the elderly.

The vestibular apparatus of the inner ear also plays a role in determining blood pressure.
• This stimulation is important to blood flow to the brain. The vestibular apparatus essentially helps us realize that we are standing up and more blood to the brain is required.

Aging is associated with loss of this vestibular stimulation and may contribute to reductions in blood flow to the brain. Thus the old adage of use it or lose it comes into play. Rock to preserve it! Let's Rock!

FURTHER BENEFITS OF THE ROCKING CHAIR

Benefits of rocking in the rocking chair also include:

- Improving the overall health of dementia patients by reducing their need for pain medication as well as lessening anxiety, depression and agitation. Study participants who rocked average of 101 minutes per day—throughout the day and not necessarily consecutively, also showed reductions in requests for pain medication. This reduction was a direct correlation with the amount of rocking. The more rocking, the greater the reduction in requests.
- Improving mood and emotional stability.

Calorie counter/metabolic primer

Another benefit of rocking may lie in the simple additional expenditure of calories. Rocking in a rocking chair is reported to double the number of calories spent compared to sitting quietly on the couch.

Expending more calories through increased activity was seen by Dr. James Levine of the Mayo Clinic as key to creating improvements in metabolism. His theory involves moving about for two additional hours a day, Therefore calories expended when using a rocking chair would benefit those who have difficulty moving. The elderly who engage in activities requiring 1,000 additional calories a day through physical activities saw significantly lessened incidences of dementia.

Active sitting: fidgeting

How many times did your mom tell you to stop fidgeting and sit still? She might have been wrong!

Fidgeting: think of it as background, subconscious movements. Research suggests fidgeting while sitting may be beneficial because it adds to the calories you are using, keeps the metabolism working and thus may be contributing to a longer life. Your mom probably did not see it this way.

Fidgeting is your body's way of telling you it wants to move but it's also a category of seated activity. You're not going anywhere but you're still moving hands or feet. Think about stretching your fingers, tapping your foot or rotating your ankles. All of these are small constant useful movements. Similarly, you could be knitting, doing self-reflexology or reading.

Doing something with your hands while seated, such as computer use, reading, knitting or driving will impact your metabolism in a more positive way than simply sitting quietly.

How does this work? Calorie expenditure is linked to metabolic function. With more calories expended there is more demand on the metabolic system. This demand interrupts the slowing down

FIDGET AWAY!

When is it socially appropriate to fidget? NEVER! But be brave. Although many people see fidgeting as a nervous behavior, just consider the time and place you fidget as a way to counteract the effects of just sitting.

At home is an easy choice. Fidget away! But what about public places? Be discrete but don't stop! Tap your foot quietly under the desk while at work.

Take notes, doodle or fidget with a pencil while stuck in a meeting. At a sporting event don't miss a chance to cheer and wave your arms in the air.

Standing and dancing is the natural act at a rock concert while actively reading the program and shouting Bravo may be all the fidgeting you can do at a classic concert program.

of the metabolism that occurs with prolonged sitting.

Without the metabolic slow down, there is an improvement in circulation and thus in the health of the blood vessels.

- Do you tap your foot as you sit? Or, do you swing your leg? If you do, you could be using 200 extra calories in two hours, according to one study. In fact, the World Health Organization recommended leg swinging and foot tapping because it was enough activity to consume excess caloric intake.
- Fidgeting your way through the day can burn up to 350 calories according to another study. When seated, tap your foot. When standing, don't just stand there, pace.
- If you can fidget while sitting by reading, working on your computer, or simply moving your hands and feet, you'll use 118 calories per hour. Compare this to the mere 80 you will burn while sitting still.
- Another study found women who fidget frequently when sitting live longer lives.
- Fidget while standing by not standing still. Instead, try walking around, answering telephones, folding sheets, interacting with a pet and you'll use 148 calories per hour. If you just stand there you will use just 87 calories per hour.

Can you even stand still for an entire hour? How long before you feel that you have to fidget?

11 Taking steps to take steps

What do we mean by taking steps? It's walking small and medium amounts of time throughout the day. This can be from two minutes to 15 minutes of activity.

Why make taking steps a part of your day? Taking steps has been shown to make a difference in weight gain and metabolism.

Is this effective? Walking around your home, office or wherever you like to ramble, is a form of low intensity physical activity. And low intensity can be all you need. With this low intensity activity, the body becomes active, the metabolism mobilizes, appetite controls are alerted, and calorie consumption increases.

The best part? Walking costs nothing and is always available as a stepping activity. No need to go anywhere special. No need to change into workout gear. No need to engage in strenuous activity. Another good thing is that counting steps is a way to track your progress. As you seek to move frequently throughout your day it will impact your weight and metabolism. You will know, step by counted step, how far you have come to your daily goal. So what is your goal? How many steps are right for you?

Walking costs nothing and is always available as a stepping activity.

In this section we'll be looking at:
• How many steps a day can help you reach your goal.
• What's the easiest way for you to measure your steps.
• How you can (painlessly) add steps to your day.

The impact on weight of taking steps

First a few facts about steps. Americans take an average of 5,117 steps a day. A desk-bound man or woman takes 5,000 to 6,000 steps a day. Each 2,000 steps taken results in an expenditure of 100 calories.

There is a relationship between weight and the number of steps taken every day:

- If you are taking fewer than 5,000 steps a day, you are considered to be embracing a sedentary or inactive lifestyle. A sedentary lifestyle is associated with weight gain.
- Taking an additional 2,000 steps throughout the day helps one maintain his or her weight. To lose weight, more steps are needed.
- Taking 7500 steps a day is the critical point for getting positive results like weight loss. In one workplace step counting program, it was found that most employees who took at least 7,500 steps a day for 16 weeks lost weight.
- Taking 8,000–10,000 steps a day promotes weight loss.
- Taking 10,000 steps a day for a year can create a significant reduction in body mass.
- In a study, it was found that taking 10,000 steps a day over eight months can result losing an average ten pounds and a decrease in waistline circumference of two inches.
- People who took 10,000 steps per day and maintained it over five years had a lower body mass index, decreased body fat, less belly fat, and better insulin sensitivity.

Yes, we are suggesting you aim at taking 10,000 steps a day. Research has shown a positive impact on weight and metabolism when you do this.

Taking 10,000 steps a day—your goal

Yes, we are suggesting you aim at taking 10,000 steps a day. Research has shown a positive impact on weight and metabolism when you do this.

Taking 10,000 steps a day has its origins with a Japanese company who wanted to promote and sell a new pedometer. This was the world's first wearable step counter and it had been invented following the 1964 Tokyo Olympics.

The idea of health as a lifestyle blossomed following these Olympic games.

Subsequently, taking 10,000 steps a day has generally been accepted as a healthy target. We really are not sure where or how the Japanese company came up with that number but it has become a daily activity recommendation. Ten thousand daily steps is now a goal endorsed by the World Health Organization, the American Heart Foundation and the US Department of Health & Human Services.

Is this a substitute for moderate exercise?

Is taking steps each day in general a substitute for the recommended 30 minutes of moderate exercise most days? The answer depends on who you ask. The general answer is, no.

Taking 10,000 steps over the course of a day is suggested in addition to a regime of moderate exercise to maintain health. However, the best strategy is do whatever you can.

Taking 10,000 steps over the course of a day is suggested in addition to a regime of moderate exercise to maintain health.

An elevated heart rate achieved through moderate exercise is a beneficial activity separate and distinct from taking steps each day. Taking 7,500 steps a day at a pace of 100 steps a minute will raise the heartbeat enough to equal 30 minutes of moderate exercise a day. Seventy five percent of Americans don't meet these exercise guidelines. If you are among them, taking steps may be an exercise option. Step yourself into that healthy 25 percent of Americans who do meet the guidelines.

The decision is yours. Do what you can—some is always better than none.

Step counters

How many steps do you take a day? How do you know? Counting steps to yourself is easy. It's also as boring as watching the proverbial paint dry. It's the Age of Technology! Use a step

FURTHER BENEFITS OF TAKING STEPS

Taking steps is known to be protective against some chronic diseases. For those with elevated risk factors, taking extra steps can cause an improvement in those risk factors.

Regular physical activity can also improve one's mental well being. It can improve sleep quality, increase concentration, reduce one's anxiety levels and is linked to a 50 percent reduction in the prevalence of depression.

Among the elderly, regular physical activity also improves cognitive and motor function. This in turn leads a 30 percent lower risk of falls.

- Taking fewer than 5,000 steps a day is associated with weight gain as well as an increase in risk of bone loss, muscle atrophy, and chronic disease.
- 6,000 total steps per day significantly reduces risk of death.
- 6,000 to 8,000 steps a day will help protect you against heart disease, stroke, various forms of cancer including breast cancer and reproductive cancers.
- If an inactive adult who takes 3,000 to 5,000 steps a day increases stepping to 7,500 to 10,000 daily steps this will improve glucose control (for those with Type 2 diabetes), lower blood cholesterol levels, and contributes to a 19 percent reduction in the risk of all-cause mortality.
- Taking 10,000 steps a day over eight months results in an average weight loss of ten pounds, decrease waistline circumference by two inches as well as a reducing high blood pressure by as much as 34 percent.
- 10,000 steps a day reduced the odds of having cardiovascular disease risk factors by 69 percent.

counter! There is a wide array of devices that can help you. There are pedometers, smart phone apps, and wearable technology such as a FitBit, VivoFit or Apple Watch. All of these will keep track of your footsteps during your day. Some cell phones apps that count steps are downloadable without cost.

Step counters are a proven incentive. Step counters keep you motivated. Studies have shown that people using step counting equipment, stay with a program of taking steps.

Caution: step counting can be addictive. One friend of ours found himself taking steps late at night in front of the water dispenser of his refrigerator. He had a few steps left to reach his goal and he wasn't going to miss out. He was determined to hit his daily goal. He knew the step counter would re-set at mid-night and go back to zero. He still had time to take 47 more steps!

Where can you walk to accumulate steps?

Anywhere. The simplest answer is around your home, office or an outside area. Author Barbara has a regular path around the living

A STEP COUNTING TIP

The Fit Bit or VivoFit fitness bands worn on the wrist use an accelerometer to count steps. Steps are counted as the arm swings. If you are not moving your arm enough, the steps will not be counted. What does this mean in practical terms? If you go shopping, you won't get credit for steps if you push the shopping cart with both hands. To get stepping credit, you can push the cart with one hand or pull the cart after you freeing the arm wearing the counting device to count steps. Or, if your hands are frequently engaged while walking like one hospital worker whose job included time spent pushing a cart with supplies, consider a step counter in necklace form.

room. Some companies have created walking lanes in their office hallways by laying down colored tape. This helps the walkers who want to take steps during breaks and lunch hours while the non walkers are not jostled by their stepping colleagues.

An important time to add steps to your day

An important time to add steps to your day is just after a meal. As noted earlier, a 10–15-minute walk helps avoid abnormal glucose levels. Fifteen to forty minutes of light intensity physical activity impacts glucose and blood sugar levels. Such activity might include walking the dog, washing your car, replacing a light bulb, cooking, raking the grass, washing dishes, ironing, and other routine or occupational tasks done while standing or walking.

Easy ways to accumulate steps in your day

It's easier than you think to add steps to your day.

First, consider how a small number of steps taken multiple times throughout the day add up. The steps you take while taking breaks from sitting are a good example. Walk for a minute and you've taken approximately 100 steps. Consider the possible number of steps you can accumulate just by stepping when you are taking hourly breaks from sitting throughout the day. They add up. You get:

- 3,200 steps a day if two-minute breaks are taken every 30 minutes over an eight-hour work day.
- 6,000 steps a day if five-minute breaks are taken each hour over 12 hours a day.
- 4,500 steps a day taking a 15-minute walk after each meal.

Tip: walk, don't run!

Add steps at a pace that's comfortable to you, take the number of steps you find easy and convenient.

Add steps at a pace that's comfortable for you, take the number of steps you find easy and convenient.

STEPS AND OBESITY

A British, radio show interviewer caught us by surprise with her question: why are Americans so fat?

It turns out where you live could very well be related to how much you weigh and how many steps a day you take. With the exception of a few big cities, America is a car nation.

We have public transportation but many of our cities are spread out, people live in the open suburbs and transportation is largely by car.

Adults in other countries use public transportation and thus walk more. They walk to get on the train, the bus and the subway and they walk after they get off the train, the bus or the subway.

One study found that people have a higher obesity rate that seems to be dependent on the average number of steps that they take each day.

In the USA, the obesity rate is 34 percent and the average daily step rate (ADSR) = 5,117.

- Australia: 16 percent obesity rate and ADSR = 9,695.
- Switzerland: 8 percent obesity rate and ADSR = 9,650.
- Japan: 3 percent obesity rate and ADSR = 7,168.

The benefits of taking the stairs

Do you live in a multi-story house or apartment building? Do you work in a multi-story office building?

If so, a calorie expending, health-improving strategy lies at your feet. Stair climbing is a form of vigorous exercise that burns more calories than jogging.

TAKING STEPS: IMPACT ON METABOLISM

Taking steps also impacts your metabolism, which has a direct connection to your weight.

10,000 steps a day

Walking 10,000 steps a day over eight months can: decrease waistline circumference by two inches, and reduce high blood pressure by 34 percent. Those who reduced their usual 10,000 steps a day to just 1,350 a day showed a definite change in just two weeks. Their metabolic rate for fats and sugars declined and their waist circumferences began increasing within two weeks.

Every 1,000 steps taken during lifestyle activities (e.g. cooking, cleaning house, mowing the lawn):

- lowers the risk of elevated waist circumference by 16 percent.
- reduces the risk of low HDL (good cholesterol) by 12 percent.
- lowers the risk of elevated triglycerides by 15 percent.
- lessens the odds of having metabolic syndrome by 13 percent.

Every 1,000 steps or every 30 minutes taken from sitting for lifestyle activities (e.g. cooking, cleaning house mowing the lawn):

- lowers the risk of elevated waist circumference by 14 percent.
- reduces the risk of low HDL (good cholesterol) by 11 percent.
- lowers the risk of elevated triglycerides by 15 percent.
- lessens the odds of having metabolic syndrome by 13 percent.

MOTIVATIONAL TIPS

Want some motivation to add steps to your day?

- Consider a competition with others. Make it a casual competition or use the feature available on many step-counting devices that allows you to compare your efforts to that of others.
- You're never wasting your time if you're moving. Step to it. Waiting for an appointment? Take steps.
- No one likes to walk in shoes that hurt their feet. Do the shoes you wear discourage you from walking? Would you walk more if your feet weren't hurting due to the shoes you wear? Is it time to go shopping?

Climbing a flight of stairs—roughly ten steps—is equivalent to taking 38 steps on level ground. That's almost four times more calories!

You might be surprised how many calories are expended using the stairs or taking the stairs instead of the elevator. StepJockey of London notes that 76 extra calories are expended when climbing up and down stairs in a five-story building twice a day and a flight of stairs to the underground/subway. This sounds small but it is powerful. The little numbers add up over time!

Each flight of stairs is calculated to expend 3.95 calories. Walking down a flight of stairs expends half that number. Consider this: just two minutes extra stair climbing a day is enough to stop average middle age weight gain. Do you have two minutes to save your life? To look better?

Step Jockey also found that maintaining one's weight is just one of the health benefits of taking the stairs.

Other positive aspects of the stair routine included improving cardiovascular fitness, protecting against high blood pressure, stopping weight gain and preventing clogged arteries.

This lowers the risk of developing chronic conditions such as diabetes, heart disease, vascular dementia and even some cancers. Bone and muscle health also improve. Thus, you end up with a lower risk of osteoporosis. Even mental health takes a turn for the better as more endorphins are released on the stair climb. https://www.stepjockey.com/health-benefits-of-stair-climbing

The benefits of cleaning house

Who ever thought cleaning house could have weight loss benefits? First, there's the calories expended. Then there's the impact on metabolism.

And a cleaner, neater environment improves your mood. How else can you regularly burn these calories?
• 15 minutes of scrubbing burns 60 calories.
• 15 minutes of vacuuming burns 50 calories.
• 30 minutes of sweeping burns 136 calories
• 60 minutes of mopping floors burns 153 calories.

Who ever thought cleaning house could have weight loss benefits?

For every 1,000 steps taken or 30 minutes of lifestyle activities of daily living (cooking, washing dishes, ironing, and other routine tasks at home or work done while standing or walking), the odds of acquiring metabolic syndrome drop by 13 percent. These are better odds than you get shooting dice in Vegas.

Improve your glucose levels by cleaning up after your meal

Taking a 15 to 40-minute walk or cleaning up for 15 to 40 minutes, after a meal, is a winning activity for one part of your metabolism. Any activity helps reduce glucose levels by 24 percent. Compare this to doing nothing but sitting for two hours after a carbohydrate rich meal. Your glucose level will not be dropping. Such a result shows a clinically significant improvement in metabolism, especially important to those who are weight challenged.

Roughly, 30 percent of overweight people are diabetic and 80 percent of diabetics are overweight.

Create active time: listening to music, watching sports, active video gaming

Pursuing your favorite activities can provide opportunities to get up and move.

Listening to music

Are you a fan of music? Why not get involved in a whole body way? Listening to music or watching a music group is a chance to get up and dance along or imitate the performers. You like air guitar? Play air guitar!

Listening to classical music is a chance to stand and conduct as the orchestra plays. It could be a chance to dust off your dancing skills and waltz or tango away.

Watching sports

Love watching those football or basketball games? Are you like a friend of ours who watches a lot of ESPN? Sports watching can add up to a lot of sitting time or it can add to your sit-less and move-more time. Why not stand up and cheer your way through the game? Prowl the living room like the coaches on the sidelines? Take a walking break during commercials?

Have some fun and lose some weight with active video gaming.

Active video gaming

Have some fun and lose some weight with active video gaming. Look what can happen! Computer programmer Mickey DeLorenzo reported he lost nine pounds and three inches from his waistline over six weeks with a 30 minutes Wii fitness regimen. The regimen included playing 15 minutes of Wii

> ## HAVE FUN!
> Active video gaming is the key to success here.
>
> Just going through the motions of playing a game doesn't do it. Get into it. Play with heart! Play with enthusiasm. Have fun!

tennis (125 calories) and 15 minutes of Wii boxing (92 calories). During these workouts, DeLorenzo emphasizes that he swung or punched, depending on the game, as hard as possible to maximize his results.

Studies on the Wii activities counted the amount of calories burned for different activities.

- Wii bowling—103 calories (average) in 30 minutes or 77 calories in 15 minutes.
- Wii baseball—70 calories (average) in 30 minutes.
- Wii boxing—92 calories in 15 minutes.
- Just Dance—200 calories (roughly) in 30 minutes.
- Wii Zumba Fitness—200–250 calories in 30 minutes.
- Guitar Hero (rock-style guitar)—204 calories in 60 minutes.
- Guitar Hero (playing drums)—272 calories in 60 minutes.

12 Your job is making you fat: here's what you can do about it

We discussed how your job was fattening you up earlier in the book. Now let's look at what you can do about it.

What can you do? What changes can be implemented by you to stop gaining weight at work because of the American workplace culture?

Build a strategy that gets you moving on the job. In this section we include:
- How to make your work life a little less convenient.
- How to take breaks from sitting.
- How your company can encourage moving more and sitting less.
- The value of sit-stand desks, standing desks.
- How office desks can encourages moving more and sitting less.
- How company-wide programs can help you.

Make your work life a little less convenient: Distance yourself from your desk.

Make your work life a little less convenient

Make your work life a little less convenient: distance yourself from your desk. Use a printer or restroom on another floor. Visit your co-worker instead of e-mailing them. (One person found there was less misunderstanding when communicating face-to-face instead of by email or text.)

Stand up to make or take phone calls. (Use a wireless headset to make it easier to walk while talking on the phone.) Stand up when anyone comes into your workspace. This reduces chatter and helps everyone get to the point more swiftly.

Take breaks from sitting

Here's the good news. Taking breaks from sitting during the workday helps you burn those calories gained by sitting still.

Take a two minute break from sitting every 20 minutes by getting up and walking.

Expending 100 calories a day can make a difference in that weight gain attributed to sitting jobs. Taking breaks also resets your metabolism.

Give your metabolism a break

Take a two-minute break from sitting every 20 minutes by getting up and walking. Even walking in place resets the metabolism. Getting up also resets the muscles, tendons and joints stretched out of place by sitting too much.

Use more calories by taking breaks

Taking multiple breaks from your office chair uses from 24 to 132 calories during the course of an eight-hour day.

The actual calories you use in a day will depend on how much of a break you take each hour:

- a one-minute break every half hour results an additional 24 calories expended.
- a two-minute break every half hour results in 59 extra calories expended.
- a five-minute break every half hour results in an 132 additional calories expended.

Tiny numbers, you might think, but remember: researchers studied how sedentary jobs contributed to weight gain in sedentary workers. Those with sitting jobs used just 100 calories less a day. By taking breaks from sitting, you can easily burn up those 100 significant calories just by standing up and moving a bit.

What happens when you take five-minute breaks from sitting every hour?

Taking breaks from sitting at work is not just about calories. Hourly five-minute breaks from sitting resulted in considerably less craving for food according to one study. Also, study volunteers reported feelings of greater happiness, less fatigue and increasing vigor throughout the day. They reported their concentration and focus was not reduced by the breaks.

Does your company encourage moving more and sitting less?

How easy is it for you to take breaks from sitting in your office? Maybe you feel awkward taking breaks from sitting. As discovered by one study, a large concern was what fellow employees might think. Will they think you're not doing your job if you're up and moving instead of sitting at your desk? This is a valid issue.

What can you do if breaks are not currently a feature at your office? It's time to create some strategies to handle this. Start slowly and quietly as you scope out the situation.

You may need to check with Human Resources to see if anything is in place. Breaks for health may be in place already. In many offices these things come and go like the seasons. There may be a workplace plan already in place but currently forgotten or disused. Find out.

• Does your office computer come equipped with a notification that it's time to stand and move? This is a good sign that someone tried to get everyone on their feet. Take advantage of the fact that, since it came with your office computer, it's work-sanctioned. (Don't disable it as did one young engineer we know.)

One of our friends worked in a break enabled office yet she didn't take breaks. Her office had a plan for breaks but it was not encouraged. She felt awkward being the only one using this office program. She began to skip her breaks. She later felt this atmosphere impacted both her weight and her health.

- Ask your HR department if the company would be interested in following the example of a Cessna factory in Wichita, Kansas. There a tone sounds at appropriate intervals to let all employees know it's time to take a break from sitting.
  Everyone knows what is happening; everyone knows why people are standing up and the awkward atmosphere vanishes.
- Casually moving about during the workday was the solution found by one friend of ours. Going to the restroom, consulting with a colleague, picking something up from a distant printer and retrieving a forgotten item from her car gave her excuses to get up and move.
- We have seen some of these strategies put to work. Our niece made it a habit when at work to always take the stairs, go to a restroom on another floor and use a printer distant from her office. Her waistlines began to shrink and no one at the office realized she was burning extra calories every day.
- Finally, instead of sitting down to solve problems with your co-worker, suggest you both walk together and talk out a solution.

Situation: everyone in the office wants to participate in a taking breaks strategy
Talk it over with your office mates and boss. You might be surprised. Some of your fellow workers may have considered moving more in the office or some may have the same weight

LOVE YOUR STAIRS!

Love your stairs! Stairs are the simplest solution. Remember that taking stairs can help you reach your step goal.

StepJockey of London noted that 76 extra calories are expended when climbing up and down stairs in a five-story building twice a day and then walking down a flight of stairs to the under ground/subway.

Those simple actions alone can burn three quarters of that 100 extra calories that help you gain weight.

and/or health concerns as you. Talk about how sitting breaks can be implemented. This will lessen the social anxiety of doing something new and different.

If everyone knows what is happening and everyone is invited and encouraged to join in, it will become the norm, not a crazy idea from that guy on the second floor. Implement some casual active ideas.

Don't just stand when taking a break. Walk in place or walk around.

Share them.
- Let everyone know you'll be using the computer stand-and-move feature. And do it.
- Set a tone heard throughout the office that lets everyone know it's time to take a break from sitting. And take the break. The tone gives everyone permission to get up and move. Hold a casual discussion and agree to how often to take a two-minute break (20 minutes, 30 minutes, hourly).
- Don't just stand when taking a break. Walk in place or walk around. And let others see you.
- Have a Fun Friday or a Wacky Wednesday. During two-minute breaks have a dance party or play balloon volleyball.
- Form an office pool to compare steps gained each day on wearable step counters.

Dove tailing interests with company health policies

Many employers are taking an interest in employee health. Does your company have a program encouraging healthy weight, blood pressure and cholesterol levels? If so, maybe you could interest your boss in instituting a stand up and move program for your workplace. Healthy employees will save the company money and improve performance. Both of these are often top of mind for company managers.

Building a healthier you should include what you do during hours at work, Let's face it, this is where you spend most of your waking hours.

ADDITIONAL BENEFITS OF TAKING BREAKS AT WORK

We have been talking about the many advantages to taking breaks from sitting for pages and pages now. How will you convince your fellow workers to take breaks with you? This question was posed to us by one reader. The talking point listed below may help you to persuade your colleagues.

- Weight gain is not the only health concern associated with more sitting time during the workday. Other changes reported in the mid-1900s, according to Men's Health, ... found that men who sat for long periods of time at work were twice as likely to develop heart disease as were men who moved around throughout the day. English bus drivers were more likely to suffer from heart attacks than bus conductors; mail sorters were more likely to suffer from heart attacks than mailmen. Definitely not good news, but probably persuasive.
- Aside from the metabolic dis-regulation potential of on-the-job sitting, pain and musculoskeletal distress are exacerbated by chair time at work. Researcher Eric Jensen notes: the typical office worker has more musculoskeletal problems than any other industry-sector worker, including construction, metal industry and transport workers. One researcher's conclusion pointed out that sitting is as much an occupational risk as lifting heavy weights on the job. (Hettinger, 1985).
- Sitting at work more than 95 percent of working time is associated with neck pain.
- Walking at work increases creativity levels during and shortly after the walk. Walkers produced twice as many creative ideas than the sitters. This is definitely a conversation starter.

ADDITIONAL BENEFITS OF TAKING BREAKS AT WORK

- Sitting on the job for ten or more years doubled the risk of colon cancer and increased the risk of rectal cancer by 44 percent.
- A Chinese study found an increased risk of ovarian cancer for women who sat at work and sat while watching television at home.
- The risk for heart attack increases by 54 percent for people who sit most of the day according to researchers at Pennington Biomedical Research Center.
- Sperm count is reduced for men who sit over two hours at a time on the job. Is everyone ready to stand up, now?

Sit-stand desks makes standing and moving easier

What if you're into your work, concentrating and not wanting to take breaks? Sit-stand desks and standing desks provide an option to conventional office desk chairs. *See* Sit-stand desks, standing desks: office desks that encourage moving more, sitting less, page 95.

Company-wide programs to help you

Company-wide policies can help you and other employees move more on the job. The resources for these policies are abundant. For example: StepJockey of London promotes use of stairs for businesses in large office buildings.

StepJockey is a digital health and property business dedicated to encouraging wellness and physical activity in the workplace. Their mission statement: we aim to label the buildings of the world for calorie burn- starting with the stairs.

StepJockey-enabled buildings allow cell phone and tablet users to download a free app to keep track of stair use. Once the app is downloaded, the user can tap or scan a Smart Sign at the start and end of each stair journey. Calories and steps are recorded and displayed. World wide team challenges are available. For a Corporate Wellness Plan, *see* https://www.stepjockey.com/health-benefits-of-stair-climbing

Check out the FitBit Corporate and their Workplace Health Programs (https://healthsolutions.fitbit.com) Create a corporate step program such as Global Corporate Challenge Pedometer Program at https://www.verywellfit.com/gcc-pedometer-program-overview-3435940

Standing meetings

Our friend was grateful to the boss who held standing meetings. Meetings became mercifully short. All cellphones, electronic devices and cups of coffee were left at the door.

Meeting participants stood during meetings. It was un-comfortable but people went straight to the items they came to discuss. Solutions were created by people who literally had both feet on the ground.

Walking meetings

Two to three people talking as they do laps along office hallways may get to be a more common sight. Such walking meetings in the workplace are shown to have physical and mental benefits as a result of being more mobile at work.

Walking people are more relaxed and generate more ideas than sitting people.

Benefits of walking meetings include:
- Accruing steps to reach a goal on wearable technology such as FitBit.
- Expending more calories (15 minutes of walking burns 56 calories while sitting at a laptop expends 20 and standing uses 22).
- Walking meeting participants are less likely to miss work for health reasons.
- Walking for as little as 15 minutes a day can add up to three years to life expectancy.
- Spurring more ideas: creative output increases by an average of

> ## KIS—KEEP IT SIMPLE
> One company created an office-walking path by sticking a line of tape down the center of the office hallway. Steppers had one lane to step and everyone else used the other lane. This made taking those important steps at the office much easier.

60 percent when people are walking.
- Walking people are more relaxed and generate more ideas than sitting people.

Tips for successful walking meetings include:
- Meet with only two or three people.
- Plan to meet for 30 minutes or less.
- Go at a speed that is comfortable for everyone so that everyone can talk.
- Walk in a park, outdoors or around the office. Inform the boss.

Walking while working

Are there other times you could walk during the workday? Certainly. Meetings, phone calls and email have come to consume more than 90 percent of the working time of managers and some other workers, such as consultants. Experts say that many of these meetings and calls could be conducted while walking.

Sit-stand desks, standing desks: office desks that encourage moving more, sitting less

Stand-able equipment for the office

Tired of sitting all day at work? Intimidated by the gym? Looking for an opportunity to expend some calories? Inspired by what you have been reading here?

You might consider a sit-stand desk or a standing desk. A sit-stand desk makes standing while you work an easy option. You can begin with the work surface placed like a regular desk. In the sit position, it is just like a regular desk. You sit and you work from a seated position. Ready to take a standing break? The desk rises up so you can go on working in a standing position.

A sit-stand desk gives you an opportunity to have an intermittent moving lifestyle at work.

You can shift from foot to foot, you can take a few fidgety steps back and forth and you can keep on working. You are stand capable. This desk will also help you to burn more calories on the job. It may even be compared to a gentle gym experience.

A sit-stand desk gives you an opportunity to have an intermittent moving lifestyle at work. You will be able to stand and work or sit and work, when you please.

Advantages: call center employees were found to be 46 percent more productive when they were stand capable, Using their sit stand desks, they stood up for an average of one and a half hours a day at work. Calories were burned, metabolisms were re-set.

A standing desk is designed to be used while standing. A high stool is frequently used for periods of sitting. It is said that Ben Franklin sometimes used a standing desk.

The jury is still out on the value of standing desks. Researchers found that just standing is not a solution to sitting too much. If you stand up, you then need to step back and forth. Continual standing can create unwanted problems such as varicose veins. For another, standing in place does not expend many more calories than sitting. Standing does not mobilize the metabolism as does walking. Stories abound of innovative companies who now have storage rooms stuffed with unused standing desks.

The standing desk is not for everyone.

On the flip side, people who have a standing desk generally rock from foot to foot, and when you're up, you inevitably walk more, Levine (a Mayo Clinic endocrinologist who is an authority on the bad effects of sitting) said. You go to the printer, you go grab some water.

There is a debate about how many calories are expended when using the sit-stand desk or standing desk at work. Various studies and various authors are writing about their different results. Among them:

• There is a 350 calories expenditure with two and a half hours of standing over an eight hour working day using a standing desk. Over ten workdays this is 3500 calories expended and the loss of one pound. By further extension, a weight loss of 20–25 pounds is anticipated over the 250 working days in a year according to researcher Dr. Mark Benden.

• Researcher Dr. John Buckley noted other benefits: 42 calories additional calories an hour are expended while standing as opposed to sitting using a sit-stand desk. By this estimate, three to four hours of standing a day results over a year in expenditure of 30,000 extra calories and the loss of eight pounds. Standing elevates the heartbeat by six to ten beats a minute. This results in increased oxygen consumption that results in increased calorie consumption. Blood glucose levels were also positively impacted by standing.

• An increased expenditure of two calories was calculated for workers standing for 15 minutes versus sitting for 15 minutes according to another study. This may account for those storerooms filled with standing desks. Researchers found that walking consumed three times as many calories as sitting or standing. The takeaway is plain—walking beat out sitting or standing still. Four 15-minute walks spaced over the day were calculated to expend 130 extra calories a day—enough to prevent weight gain.

One small study showed 100 extra calories were expended during an hour of use at a treadmill desk.

The treadmill desk

The treadmill desk pairs a treadmill with an appropriately situated work surface/desk. You walk and you work. One small study showed 100 extra calories were expended during an hour of use at a treadmill desk. The speed was slow, just one mile per hour.

Users like the idea of dual purposing work and exercise. One company now holds walking meetings—on treadmills. Using two treadmill desks facing two other treadmill desks, the participants can talk and walk. The company also has a room with six treadmill desks that their employees can use whenever they wish.

Employees at a US Air Force facility found it difficult to stay awake during boring, night shifts. Using a treadmill desk helped keep everyone awake.

The advantage of the treadmill desk is one of a healthy work environment. The drawbacks include expense and the bulky size that requires big workspaces. Treadmill desks are definitely something that should be tried before committing to installation and purchase.

The exercise ball chair/office chair

Sitting on an exercise ball burns four more calories an hour than sitting in a chair. This is about 30 extra calories burned in a workday.

Maintaining balance as one sits on an exercise ball requires minute muscular adjustments and engages the postural muscles. It takes a bit of practice. Research finds that sitting on the exercise balls increases blood circulation up and down the spinal column and to the brain. This increased circulation in turn oxygenates the blood the brain receives.

UNDER-DESK CYCLE CONSIDERATIONS

Questions to be considered when shopping for an under-desk cycle (according to Weight Loss Resources Limited).

1. How much noise would be created by the under desk cycle?
2. Will it fit under your desk with your legs moving?

Active sitting on the job, the under-desk cycle

As noted earlier, fidgeting and rocking while seated helps to burn calories and reset the metabolism. But fidgeting and rocking can hardly compare to using the under-desk bicycle (really!). Yes, there really is such a thing as the under-desk bicycle. This under-the-desk device was designed to move the legs in a cycling motion.

Using an under-desk cycle at work helped one group of study participants to lose weight and waistline. Pedaling when they choose, group members expended an average of 107 extra calories a day. Over 16 weeks they experienced beneficial changes in weight, total fat mass, body fat percentage, and resting heart rate.

The number of minutes of cycling a day was associated with improved performance at work.

These outcomes were accomplished as study participants peddled under their desks on 70 percent of workdays. They peddled for 50 minutes a day in sessions lasting an average of four and a half minutes. An average of 18 times a day participants were pedaling away at approximately 60 rpm.

How do you make this work for you? According to the study, if it is weight loss you're after then by spending more time pedaling and having more separate pedaling sessions per day and per week, you will increase your calorie burn, decrease your body fat, lose more weight and improve your resting heart rate. The quicker the pedaling speed, the significantly greater the decrease in waistline.

The number of minutes of cycling a day was associated with improved performance at work. This including better concentration and fewer days missed because of physical or mental health problems.

Part four

YOUR INTERMITTENT MOVING LIFESTYLE WEIGHT LOSS PLAN

13 Planning a weight loss lifestyle

You've read about strategies to move more and sit less. Now it's time to create your own, unique intermittent moving plan. And time is what it's all about.

Your plan is about when and where you intend to add more moving time and create less sitting time to your day and evening. The key to the success here is creating a new habit and a new lifestyle. As suggested by many experts, give yourself 21 days. That's how long it takes to effectively form any habit. That's the amount of time needed for the brain to change.

You'll find moving more, sitting less goes from a conscious effort to a subconscious effort. After awhile you just know you've been sitting too long. It will become intuitive. You won't even need a clock to remind you to move.

How long before you see results from your efforts? There is no answer to that question. Everyone is different in terms of past activity. Everyone is different in applying an intermittent moving plan. In general, those who have been the least active in the past and those who become the most active in the present will see the most results. As Kevin says, "Move more to lose more."

Central to your success are two pieces of equipment: a timer and a step counter.

Getting started

Central to your success are two pieces of equipment: a timer and a step counter. This is how you'll be measuring the doses of moving more and sitting less that will help you to achieve your goals.

BE YOUR OWN BODY MANAGER

Remember: for every individual an opportunity exists to move deliberately through the day. This will influence his or her weight. Your role is be a body manager; to create the timing of sitting, standing and moving activities to keep your metabolism operating as it should, to signal your appetite control system and to maintain expenditure of calories so they match and surpass calorie consumption.

Decide which device, a cell phone or a kitchen timer will work best for each of your moving and sitting situations. Next, invest in a device to count your steps. Look for a wearable step counter, a Smart Watch or download the appropriate app for your smart phone.

Begin your intermittent moving efforts by observing your usual habits. Using your step counter track the steps you take on a normal day. Also, follow your sitting habits. Have a piece of paper and your timer handy. Just as you would with a food diary, write down how long you sit at any one time and how often you get up and move during an hour. This baseline will give you an idea of your usual activity level.

Make this the first entry in your move more, sit-less diary. Keep track of your on-going efforts. Create space to note 21 days of activity. At the end of each day, summarize what you've accomplished throughout that day. Write down the total number of steps you've taken that day and the total number of breaks from sitting.

Remember you want to shoot for 10,000 steps and 16 breaks. You are now on your way! Good Luck, Bon voyage and have a fun time!

14 Your move more, sit less plan

Two basic plans are presented here. Choose one and try it out. If you are dissatisfied, try the other one. It's your choice.

One includes more frequent breaks from sitting. Use these as goals. Be realistic. This is a new life style, a new way of looking at things. There is a period of adjustment. Some days you will be more successful at following the plan than other days. Becoming accustomed to taking breaks and increasing your number of steps will take time.

Be patient with yourself. You may discover you need a new pair of comfortable walking shoes. You may want a thermal coffee cup to use while you take your walking coffee break. You may need to get up earlier in the morning.

You can figure this out.

Plan one
- Take breaks from sitting, getting up every 20 to 30 minutes and moving around for two minutes throughout the day and evening.
- Take a 15-minute walk (around the house or office or outdoors) after each meal.
- Accumulate 10,000 steps a day.
- Use active sitting ideas in the evening.

Plan Two

- Take breaks from sitting, getting up every hour and moving around for five minutes throughout the day and evening.
- Take a 15-minute walk (around the house or office; outdoors) after each meal.
- Accumulate 10,000 steps a day.
- Implement active sitting ideas in the evening.

Writing your intermittent moving plan

Now make your plan. Consider when and where during your day you have an opportunity to move more and sit less. Set some goals. Write it down. Now try it out.

Now make your plan. Consider when and where during your day you have an opportunity to move more and sit less.

Morning

Getting moving. You've had breakfast and it's time for a 15-minute walk around the house, outdoors or as part of your commute to the office.

Keep moving at the office. Plan your breaks from sitting: how to time them, when to take them, ways to take them. (*See* pages 93–99 for tips.) Be creative in your approach.

Keep moving if you spend your day at home. Plan your breaks from sitting: how will you time them, when will you take them?

Have your daily goals in mind. For example, how many steps do you want to take by noon?

Noon

Lunch break at the office or home. Make plans where to walk for 15 minutes after eating. Where will you go?

Afternoon

Keep moving. Continue your breaks from sitting. How many breaks can you take? How many steps have you accumulated? (*See* page 80 for tips.)

Evening

After dinner, be thoughtful. Avoid the nightly collapse! Make plans to walk for 15 minutes after eating. Where will you go?

Your evening includes a lot of potential time for your benefit, roughly four to five hours before you go to bed. Keep moving. Take breaks from sitting. Sit actively. Be active while watching television, texting, or using social media or do something active such as pursuing a hobby, playing with your children or pets, cleaning house, or exercising.

Do remember to write in your plan and summarize your day before you go to bed.

Evaluate your plan

How did your plan work? Are you happy with it? Are you moving more and sitting less than you did previously?

Do you think your plan needs work? Don't hesitate to makes changes. Find what works for you. Is motivation or finding time that a challenge? For tips on motivation, *see* page 83. For tips on finding time, *see* Found time, page 109.

Did you move toward the number of steps and breaks that you set as a goal?

15 Fitting something new into your lifestyle

Lifestyles vary. If your day is spent in one of the following ways, here are some tips to accommodate your day and evening to create a weight loss

You're on your feet moving all day at work. You accumulate a lot of steps on the job. Watch out for the nightly collapse. In the evening you'll want to put Plan One into play.

You're on your feet standing all day at work. Remember: while standing you expend only a few calories more than when you sit. As you stand, shift your weight from foot to foot. Walk in place when you can. Walk whenever you can on the job. Add steps during breaks and lunch, before work and in the evening. *See* Make your work life a little less convenient, page 87.

You sit behind the wheel of a vehicle all day. Maybe you are making sales calls or deliveries; maybe you drive a bus, taxi, Lyft or Uber. Find time during the day to add steps, Can you get out of your car and stand while you are waiting on a client?

Can you stand up during your lunch hour? Can you park in the most distance parking space at scheduled stops? Will you remember to use the stairs whenever possible? *See* Found time, page 109.

Watch out for the nightly collapse. In the evening you'll want to put Plan One into play.

You have difficulty moving. As much as you'd like to add steps or take breaks from sitting, you have difficulty moving or getting up from a seated position. Active sitting may be for you. The rocking chair is your friend. *See* Fidgeting, pages 72–73.

Creating success
Take the first step.
1. Make the active, conscious decision you're going to work at being aware of how much you sit, stand and move.
2. Be aware. Be aware of how long you sit, stand or move. Be aware of how often you move. Remember: it's all about time and timing.

Consider: what is success? Success is many things. For Kevin success was being in control of his weight and his body. For some success is making the effort to move more, sit less. For others it's about weight loss. Once you make an effort and see some success, you'll want to move more.

Celebrate your success! Give yourself a pat on the back. Every single step counts and its appreciated by your body. Every step is a step in the right direction. Every step can change metabolism. Tell yourself, Good job! Congratulate yourself for what you're doing: leaving your comfy chair behind, taking a break from sitting, walking for two minutes or 15. Keep going. Every step carries you closer to your goal. You're setting the scene for taking control of your body. What you're doing is having an impact.

Every step can change metabolism. Tell yourself, Good job!

Your thoughts are things. Keep them positive. You are unstoppable. You can change your metabolism. There's only one person who can stop you.

Be consistent. Consistency is the key to success. Moving consistently throughout your day helps maintain a natural balance in your metabolism. According to researchers, intermittent moving throughout the 16 hours you're awake is important. It's more important than 30 minutes of exercise.

Make extra copies of your written plan. Station them where you sit and read them every day. Write down your goals: weight loss, waistline loss, better energy. Whatever gives you motivation. All of this will make it become more real.

Living your plan: making your body your hobby
Found time
Do you feel there's just no time in your day to add more moving? Consider found time. You slightly change what you're doing. Our

TIPS TO KEEP MOVING

- Park farther out in any parking lot
- Use the stairs when available. If you have to go up three flights of stairs but you can only manage one flight, then walk up one and take the elevator for the next two.
- Convert the activities you do while sitting, into something you do standing or walking. You can use social media or video gaming. Create a standing platform so you can play your game on your device or laptop while standing up.
- Sit actively. Sit in a rocking chair so you can rock. Do more than just watch the television: rock, knit, read, or tap your foot.
- Make a game of it. Challenge yourself to add steps and breaks from sitting to your day and evening. See how many ways you can prompt yourself to stand and move.
- Get creative. It's a challenge to break up your pattern of sitting. It's critical to put in the time to move. While traveling, you could take laps of the terminal. Take steps in your hotel room while you unpack. When possible, walk to events. Do sightseeing on foot. Take the stairs. Take the steps.

friend, a pharmaceutical saleswoman, for example, spends her working days in an SUV all day traveling from dental office to dental office. Her found time strategy? Parking in the parking place furthest from the door. Taking the stairs whenever possible.

You can use previously sedentary time as moving time:
- Move about during coffee breaks or at lunch. Stand up every time you talk on the phone. Stand up every time someone comes into your work area. Stand up every time you speak to someone at work.
- Be mindful. Value the time when you are moving. Value the time spent commuting to work by public transportation. Give up your seat to someone weary and fat!
- During time spent on the phone, texting or on social media, move or step in place. Swing your arms. Gesture broadly with your entire body. Place your phone at a convenient standing height to free your hands and arms.
- Take advantage of time spent waiting: look at all the time you have between work appointments, waiting for a personal appointment, waiting in line. (You actually don't have to sit down in a waiting room!). Toe tapping while waiting or seated during meetings is a possibility.

This is what found time is all about. Are there more opportunities in your day for finding found time? (*See* Active sitting: fidgeting, page 72).

16 Making your plan work

Identify hot spots—where do you sit? What is your regular sitting spot? Is it possibly a hot spot for sitting too much? This is where you will accumulate your sitting time. Identify it. Recognize it. Change it.

Station reminders there to move. Place a timing device, your kitchen timer or cell phone there so you can time yourself. Stick a Post-It in sight as reminder to move a certain time. Put them on the television, the computer screen or the gaming controller.

Create triggers

Create triggers. Look for your own triggers. What prompts you to sit? Is it reading the paper? Working the Sudoku? Watching a certain television program? What will trigger you to move? Use them.

Timers are one form of a trigger. Notes posted where you will see them as you sit is another. After awhile you wont need reminders. You'll just know when it's time to move.

Choose what works for you

You'll want to choose what works for you, what moving more habits fit you and your life. If it works and you like it, you'll be more likely to continue doing it.

If you find yourself not moving more and sitting less, it's time to re-evalute.

If you find yourself not moving more and sitting less, it's time to re-evaluate. What changes could you make to get yourself moving towards your goals?

Make a pact with family or friends

A common problem to an intermittent moving plan is overcoming society's pressure to sit. Make a pact with family and friends. As you're sitting around socializing, let them know you'll be getting up and taking a break from sitting every 20–25 minutes.

Does anyone need anything? You can ask as you stand up and move. And why not invite them to get up and move too?

The re-set button

Maybe today didn't work particularly well. Maybe you couldn't make good on your intentions to move. Forgive yourself for falling off the wagon. Remember that this is a process. This is where the re-set button comes in. Just restart. Tomorrow's another day.

Just start the day thinking positively. Some days it's harder than others to make this habit work. Let gentle guilt work for you but remember: positive action is the key to stimulate rebooting.

Let gentle guilt work for you but remember: positive action is the key to stimulate rebooting.

Bribe yourself

Use rewards.

Make your goal on one day and celebrate! Dance to your favorite music. Be silly. Put stars all over that page of your movement diary. Gone through a whole day following your moving more, sitting-less plan? Figured out how to move more at work? Good job!. A reward is in order.

You decide when a reward is earned and what the reward is. Maybe you'll reward yourself with vivid mental images of reaching your goal. Maybe you will go outside and play a game of hopscotch.

It's all up to you.

Troubleshooting

Have you talked yourself out of moving? Are you having a hard time getting into the habit of getting up and moving more?

Maybe you're talking yourself out of moving. Listen to yourself.

Maybe you're talking yourself out of moving. Listen to yourself. What internal conversation are you having about moving or not moving? How do you talk yourself out of moving?

I don't feel like moving, getting up from my comfy chair.
I'm so tired. I've been on my feet all day
My feet hurt. My back hurts. My knees hurt.

Does this sound familiar? Do your internal conversations that keep you from moving sound like this?
• Do you use a delaying tactic?
  I'll get up in a little bit.
• I'm too busy to leave my chair.
  I have to finish my work. I'm on a deadline.
• It's how I work. This is how I concentrate.
  I will just buckle down and in four hours I'll be done and then
  I'll get up and move.
• I can't stop playing.
• I don't need to move.
• I'll move more later today.

Then there's the recruiting others tactic where you get others to move for you:
Would you get that for me?
While you're up, would you do this for me?

Are you literally talking yourself out of moving? We know about it. We've done it. Guess what? While you're having this conversation with yourself, your body's going about its job. It's shutting down all sorts of metabolic activities.

There is, of course, a price to be paid. Here's the guilt trip part of our message. Have you heard the old saying? Enjoy now, pay later? Whatever energy saving you think you are doing or what other purpose you're serving by sitting now, there is a greater price to be paid later in weight gain and health concerns.

What's your motivation strategy?

What's your motivation strategy for following your plan? How do you get yourself up and get moving enough to trim that waistline and impact your weight?

Playing a game

Make it game. Can you succeed at taking the breaks you want every day? Can you walk for 15 minutes after each meal? Can you use a step counter to take a certain number of steps? Make it a game. Keep a scorecard.

Do you have friends or family members who would like to work toward weight loss goals and would be interested in making a game of comparing step count numbers? Stand up and call them up and start playing!

Count moving calories

Some people lose weight by counting the number of calories in what they eat. Why not count the calories you spend while moving? If you're not moving, you're not spending the calories you could. It's time to think about moving and spending those calories.

Remember, getting up and moving is worth calories. In an eight-hour workday, a one-minute break from sitting every half hour results in the expenditure of an additional 24 calories. A two-minute break every half hour results in 59 extra calories spent. A five-minute break every half hour results in 132 additional calories expended. Can you see where this is going? For more calorie counting numbers, *see* Counting calories expended, pages 117–120.

Remember, getting up and moving is worth calories.

Motivation: this is free

Many weight loss programs and strategies cost money. This is free.

Think about the things you have to do. It's always about time, money and effort: how much time does it take; how much money does it cost and how much effort is needed.

Intermittent moving doesn't take much time and it's free.

Intermittent moving doesn't take much time and it's free. It is all about effort. It's about what the body reads as motion. It's about giving your body what it needs to be healthier, thinner, stronger.

Motivation: accentuate the positives

If you want to succeed in weight loss, focus on the positives. Here's some of the positives you can tell yourself as you move your way to success.

If you want to succeed in weight loss, focus on the positives.

- Moving is a path to success: moving is success in weight loss. Moving is success at waist loss.
- What you do today matters tomorrow. It's not just weight control, it's overall well-being, both physical and mental.
- You're reshaping your body and sharpening your mind.
- Others have done this and succeeded.
- Every single footstep makes a difference.
- Every move you make; every step you take is creating the reality you want.
- All that weight you've tried to take off and never lost, here's the potential for a slim, trim you.
- You're not only succeeding at weight control, you're showing you're in control.
- You're lessening your risk for a host of future ills.
- This is about empowerment. This is about taking control when you've felt out of control for so many years.
- If you're consistent at this, you're going to change.
- Mindfulness is focus. Focus on movement: when you stand, when you move, how much and how often.

- Yes, you can lose weight. Yes, you can be more energetic. Your ideal, can you reach it? Yes, you can.
- This isn't adding something to your day: it's doing it a different way.
- Appreciate what you've done.
- Believe it's making a difference.

Appendix and summaries

Strategies to trim your waistline
Are you concerned about the size of your waistline? Do you even know where it is? Doctors do. They measure two inches below the bellybutton.

There is reason to focus on your waistline. Elevated waist circumference is an indicator for cardiovascular disease, stroke, heart attack, cognitive decline, Alzheimer's disease, cancer, obesity and metabolic syndrome.

The more you sit, the bigger your waistline. For example, men who sit more than four hours per day during their time off from work, have almost double the chances for a bigger waistline. Reaffirm your decision to move more and sit less by considering how your waistline is impacted.

Here's the plan. Measure your waistline. Write it down. Now forget it. Move on. You can check it again when your pants fall off.

Take breaks from sitting
Taking breaks from sitting has more impact on waistline size than exercise. Those who take the most breaks in sitting have smaller waistlines by an average of 1.6 inches.

Take 10,000 steps a day
Walking 10,000 steps a day over eight months can decrease waistline circumference by two inches.

Light intensity physical activity
Being active around the house or office impacts your waistline. Things like cooking, washing dishes, taking out the trash, feeding the dog, ironing, cleaning sand other routine domestic or occupational tasks done while standing or walking are forms

of light exercise. Results of one study showed every 1,000 steps taken during such light intensity physical activity reduced the risk of elevated waist circumference by16 percent.

Counting calories expended

If you're counting the calories of the food you eat, why not count the calories you use as you move? Consider how what you do during the day translates into calorie expenditure.

If you're counting the calories of the food you eat, why not count the calories you use as you move?

When you are taking steps every 2,000 steps (roughly a mile): equals 100 calories used. When you take 10,000 steps a day you use up 500 calories. (for a 180 pound person) If you use 500 extra calories a day, you will lose a pound in a week!

Calories: sitting, standing, moving

- Lying down for an hour uses 77 calories.
- Sitting for an hour uses 75 calories.
- Standing for an hour uses 84 calories.
- Moving for an hour uses 150 calories.
- Sitting while fidgeting for an hour uses 118 calories.
- Standing while fidgeting (walking around, answering telephones, changing a video, folding sheets, interacting with a pet) uses 148 calories per hour.

Rocking calories

Rocking in a rocking chair uses 150 calories per hour.

Taking breaks from sitting

Over an eight-hour work day:

- A one-minute break taken from sitting every half hour results in the expenditure of an additional 24 calories.
- A two-minute break every half hour results in 59 extra calories expended
- A five-minute break every half hour results in an 132 additional calories expended.

Calories expended taking stepping breaks during commercials

- You will use 148 calories for every 2,000 steps you take during your television commercials. If you watch television for an hour, there will be 16 to 24 minutes of commercials in one hour.
- This is 79 calories more that will be burned if you watched television for an hour and remained sitting.

Calorie-using opportunities around the house

Reward yourself with the mindful thought that you're expending calories as you work around the house. The National Institute of Health has figured it out for us. Below is a calories expended count for a 150 pound person measured in 30 minute increments.

- Vacuuming 84 calories.
- Washing dishes 76 calories.
- Doing laundry 72 calories.
- Scrubbing floors 189 calories.
- Gardening 162 calories
- Cleaning windows 153 calories.
- Playing with a dog 115 calories per hour.
- Chasing after kids 120 calories per hour.
- Walking in park 130 calories per hour.
- Mall type shopping 135 calories per hour.
- Driving a vehicle 120 calories per hour.

Calories expended during a typical day at the office

Below are two ways to spend calories during your day at the office. With a little planning, you can change your routine and up your calorie use. (Adapted from *Move a Little, Lose a Lot* by Dr. James Levine and Selene Yeager)

- Park by close to your office building, and take the elevator to your floor: 15 calories
  Or
  Park five blocks from office. Take stairs to your floor: 80–120 calories.
- Make phone calls for an hour at your desk: 15 calories

Or
Take calls standing up and pacing with notepad on bookcase
or filing cabinet to take notes without bending down: 100–130
calories.

• Take a seated 45-minute lunch: 25 calories.
Or
Walk for 30 minutes at lunch; sitting and eating for 15 minutes:
100–130 calories.

• Stay seated during a one-shour meeting: 15 calories.
Or
Walk for one hour during a one hour walking meeting: 150–200
calories.

• Take the elevator to ground floor and walk to your car parked
close to the building. Drive home: 15 calories.
Or
Take stairs out of the building, walk back to car parked in a
distant parking spot 80–100.

The choice is yours. Use a total of 85 calories or use a total of
510–680 calories.

Calories expended using a standing desk at the office
According to Dr. Mark Benden, researcher and author of *Could
You Stand to Lose*, using a standing desk in the office offers an
opportunity to lose weight.

Standing burns 40 percent more calories than
sitting, which translates to weight loss for a 175
pound person in the following way:

*Standing burns 40
percent more calories
than sitting*

• Standing for two and a half hours each day would
result in an extra energy expenditure of 350 calories per day.
• It takes 3,500 calories to equal 1 pound of weight loss.
• Ten days of 350 calories per day equals one pound of weight loss.
• There are 250 working days in a year or the potential for 20–25
pounds of weight loss in a year by adopting this method of working.

Standing desk or sit-stand desk (Alternate calorie estimate)

Another view for the calorie count of using a standing desk calculated by comparing numerous studies found standing for 6 hours during the work day resulted in 54 additional calories expended. That's 270 calories used up in a workweek.

Bibliography

Bachman, Rachel, "The office walk-and-talk really works," *Wall Street Journal*, Sept. 12, 2016

Carr, Lucas J.; Leonhard, Christoph; Tucker, Sharon; Fethke, Nathan; Benzo, Roberto; Gerr, Fred, "Total Worker Health Intervention Increases Activity of Sedentary Workers," *American Journal of Preventive Medicine* 2015; DOI: 10.1016/j.amepre.2015.06.022

Ching, Pamela L.YH ScD, RD; Wilet, Walter C., MD; Rimm, Eric B., ScD; Colditz, Graham A. MBBS; Gotmaker, Steven L., PhD; and Stampfer, Meir J., MD, "Activity Level and Risk of Overweight in Male Health Professionals," *American Journal of PublicHealth*, January 1996, Vp;. 86, No. 1

Church, TS; Thomas, DM; Tudor-Locke C; Katzmarzyk PT; Earnest CP; Rodarte RQ; Martin CK; Blair SN; Bouchard C, "Trends over 5 decades in U.S. occupation-related physical activity and their associations with obesity," PLoS One. 2011;6(5):e19657. doi: 10.1371/journal.pone. 0019657. Epub 2011 May 25.

Dunstan DW, Kingwell BA, Larsen R, Healy GN, Cerin E, Hamilton MT, Shaw JE, Bertovic DA, Zimmet PZ, Salmon J, Owen N, "Breaking Up Prolonged Sitting Reduces Postprandial Glucose and Insulin Responses." *Diabetes Care*, 2012 Feb 28.

Dunstan, David W. PhD, BAppSc; "Screen-based Entertainment Time, All-cause Mortality, and Cardiovascular Events: Population-based Study With Ongoing Mortality and Hospital Events Follow-up," *Journal of the American College of Cardiology*, 2011;57(3):292-299.

Healy GN; Dunstan DW; Salmon J, et al., "Breaks in sedentary time: Beneficial associations with metabolic risk.," *Diabetes Care*, 2008;31:661–666.

Dos Santos, Hildemar MD, DrPH, Dinhluu Bredehoft, Margaret MPH, DrPH, Gonzalez, Frecia M. MPH, "Exercise Video Games and Exercise Self-Efficacy in Children," *Global Pediatric Health*, April 26, 2016, 3: 2333794X16644139.

Heid, Markham, "The Case For Taking a Walk After You Eat." *Time Health*, September 26, 2018 Page 1_ 14 of 1_ 22

Hellmich, Nanci, "Q&A: How to drop pounds with all-day activities, not exercise," *USA Today*, January 21, 2009

Hu FB, Li TY, Colditz GA, Willett WC, Manson JE. Television watching and other sedentary behaviors in relation to risk of obesity and type 2 diabetes mellitus in women. JAMA 2003;289:1785–1791

Judson, Olivia, "Stand Up While You Read This!" February 23, 2010, http:// opinionator. blogs.nytimes.com/2010/02/23/stand-up-while-you-read-this/?hp.

Katzmarzyk, Peter T., "Physical Activity, Sedentary Behavior, and Health: Paradigm Paralysis or Paradigm Shift?," *Diabetes*, 2010 Nov;59(11):2715-6.PMID: 2098047

Katzmarzyk, Peter T. Ph.D., "Leisure Time Sedentary Behavior, Occupational/Domestic Physical Activity, and Metabolic Syndrome in U.S. Men and Women," Metab Syndr Relat Disord. 2009 December; 7(6): 529–536. doi: 10.1089/met.2009.0023 PMCID: PMC2796695 NIHMSID: NIHMS132193

Kunz, Barbara and Kevin, *Un-Sit Your Life, The Reflex "Diet" Solution, Change your sitting habits, empower your life*, RTS Publishing, 2015

Levine JA, Schleusner SJ, Jensen MD., "Energy expenditure of nonexercise activity," Am J Clin Nutr 2000;72:1451–1454.

Mclean L, Tingley M, Scott RN, Rickards J., "Computer terminal work and the benefit of microbreaks," Appl Ergon. 2001 Jun;32(3):225-37. Page 1_ 15 of 1_ 22

Nygaard H, Tomten SE, Høstmark AT., "Slow postmeal walking reduces postprandial glycemia in middle-aged women." Appl Physiol Nutr Metab. 2009 Dec;34(6):1087-92

Ojeda-Zapata, Julio, "Desk Jockeys Stand Up to Work on Getting More Fit," *Pioneer Press*, January 10, 2015.

Painter, Kim, Your Health: Too much sitting puts the body on idle, *USA Today*, 1/31/2010

Patel, Alpa V., Bernstein, Leslie, Deka, Anusila, Feigelson, Heath Spencer, Campbell, Peter T., Gapstur, Susan M., Colditz, Grahan A., and Thun, Michael J., "Leisure Time Spent Sitting in Relation to Total Mortality in a Prospective Cohort of US Adults." Am J Epid Published online July 22, 2010 (DOI: 10.1093/aje/kwq155)

Reddy, Sumathi, "Hard Math: Adding Up Just How Little We Actually Move," **Wall Street Journal**, Your Health, March 11, 2013

Reynolds, Gretchen, "Does Fidgeting Counter Harmful Effects of Sitting?, Any movement, no matter how slight, counts as physical activity and can be good for your health," *New York Times*, July 20, 2018

Reynolds, Gretchen, "Get Up! Stand Up!" *New York Times*, Sept. 13, 2017

Reynolds, Gretchen, "How Our Bones Might Help Keep Our Weight in Check," *New York Times*, Jan. 17, 2018

Reynolds, Gretchen, "How many calories we burn when we sit, stand, walk," *New York Times*, June 22, 2016

Reynolds, Gretchen, "A Sprained Ankle May Have Lifelong Consequences, *New York Times*, September 16, 2015

Reynolds, Gretchen, "Work. Walk 5 minutes, Work." *New York Times*, December 28, 2016

Salmon J, Bauman A, Crawford D, Timperio A, Owen N. "The association between television viewing and overweight among Australian adults participating in varying levels of leisure-time physical activity," Int J Obes Relat Metab Disord 2000;24:600–606

Shea, Christopher, "Mindful Exercise," *New York Times*, Dec. 9, 2007

Shields M, Tremblay MS, "Sedentary behavior and obesity," *Health Rep*, 2008 Jun: 19(2): 19–30

Stamatakis, Emmanuel Anne, PhD, MSc, BSc; Hamer, Mark PhD, MSc, BSc; Dunstan, David W. PhD, BAppSc; "Screen-based Entertainment Time, All-cause Mortality, and Cardiovascular Events: Population-based Study With Ongoing Mortality and Hospital Events Follow-up," Journal of the American College of Cardiology. 2011;57(3):292-299.

Steeves JA, Thompson DL, Bassett DR Jr., "Can sedentary behavior be made more active? A randomized pilot study of TV commercial stepping versus walking," Med Sci Sports Exerc. 2012 Feb;44(2):330-5. doi: 10.1249/MSS.0b013e31822d797e.

Stein, Rob, "Fidgeting Helps Separate the Lean From the Obese, Study Finds," *Washington Post*, January 28, 2005; Page A02 Page 1_ 17 of 1_ 22

Sisson, Susan B. Ph.D., Camhi, Sarah M. Ph.D., Church, Timothy S. M.D., M.P.H., Ph.D., Martin, Corby K. Ph.D., Tudor-Locke, Catrine

Ph.D., Bouchard, Claude Ph.D., Earnest, Conrad P. Ph.D., Smith, Steven R. M.D., Newton, Jr., Robert L. M.D., Rankinen, Tuomo Ph.D., and Katzmarzyk, Peter T. Ph.D., "Leisure Time Sedentary Behavior, Occupational/Domestic Physical Activity, and Metabolic Syndrome in U.S. Men and Women," Metab Syndr Relat Disord. 2009 December; 7(6): 529–536. doi: 10.1089/met.2009.0023 PMCID: PMC2796695 NIHMSID: NIHMS132193

Thomee, Sara; Lissner, Lauren; Hagberg, Mats; Grimby-Ekman, Anna, "Leisure Time Computer Use and Overweight Development in Young Adults – A Prospective Study," *BMC Public Health*, 2015;15(839)

Vlahos, James, "Is Sitting a Lethal Activity?," *The New York Times Magazine*, April 14, 2011

"Foreign Exchange," *Women's Health*, March 2011, p. 26

Steeves, Jeremy Adam, Bassett, David. Fotzhugh, Eugene c., Thompson, Dixie, L., "Can sedentary behavior be made more active? A randomized pilot study of TV commercial stepping versus walking," *International Journal of Behavioral Nutrition and Physical Activity*, 9(1): 95, August 2012

Tucker LA, Bagwell M. Television viewing and obesity in adult females. Am J Public Health 1991;81:908–911

Tucker LA, Friedman GM. "Television viewing and obesity in adult males." Am J Public Health 1989;79:516–518 Abstract/ Page 1_18 of 1_22

Vandelanotte C, Sugiyama T, Gardiner P, Owen N., "Associations of leisure-time internet and computer use with overweight and obesity, physical activity and sedentary behaviors: crosssectional study," J Med Internet Res. 2009 Jul 27;11(3):e28

Vlahos, James, "Is Sitting a Lethal Activity?," *The New York Times Magazine*, April 14, 2011

Links

Arney, Katharine, "TV watching 'makes you obese'," BBC News, 22 April, 2003, http://news.bbc.co.uk/2/hi/health/2966843.stm

Cox, David, "Watch your step: why the 10,000 daily goal is built on bad science," The Guardian, Sept. 3, 2018, https://www.theguardian.com/lifeandstyle/2018/sep/03/watch-your-step-why-the-10000-daily-goal-is-built-on-bad-science

Ferreri, Deana, "Stand up, walk around, and cut down on inflammation," February 16, 2011, http://yummyplants.com/vegan-nutrition/stand-up-walk-around-cut-down-on-inflammation/

"Fidgeting feet: An annoying habit that's good for you?," Japan Today, Oct. 27, 2015, https://japantoday.com/category/features/kuchikomi/fidgeting-feet-an-annoying-habit-thats-good-for-you

Klein, Sarah, "The Surprising Number of Steps Americans Really Take Each Day," July 13, 2017, https://www.health.com/fitness/number-of-steps-americans-take-daily

Levine, James A., "Sitting down is KILLING you! Heart disease, obesity, depression and crumbling bones—a terrifying new book by a top doctor reveals they are all linked to the hours we spend in chairs," 25 July 2014, https://www.dailymail.co.uk/news/article-2706317/Sitting-KILLING-Heart-disease-obesity-depression-crumbling-bones-terrifying-new-book-doctor-reveals-linked-hours-spend-chairs.html

Mann, Denise, "Taking 10,000 Steps a Day May Lower Diabetes Risk: Study Shows Building Up to 10,000 Steps a Day May Lead to Weight Loss and Better Insulin Sensitivity," Jan. 14, 2011, https://www.webmd.com/diabetes/news/20110113/taking-10000-steps-a-day-may-lower-diabetes-risk#1

Mason, Emma, "Study finds more breaks from sitting are good for waistlines and hearts," 11 Jan 2011, https://www.eurekalert.org/pub_releases/2011-01/esoc-sfm010911.php

McDowell, Dena, "How many steps per day to lose weight?" https://www.livestrong.com/article/171629-how-many-steps-per-day-to-lose-weight/

Miller, Kelli, "Active' Video Games Burn Calories Study: Kids Who Play Active Video Games Burn Four Times as Many Calories as Kids Who Play Traditional Games", https://www.webmd.com/children/news/20080902/active-video-games-burn-calories

Schulte, Brigid, "Health experts have figured out how much time you should sit each day," Washington Post, 2 June 2015, https://www.washingtonpost.com/news/wonk/wp/2015/06/02/medical-researchers-have-figured-out-how-much-time-is-okay-to-spend-sitting-each-day/?utm_term=.7e990ad069b3

Spalding, Anne, Kelly, Linda, "Rewards for Using Exercise Balls." (Excerpt from Fitness on the Ball), https://us.humankinetics.com/blogs/excerpt/rewards-for-using-exercise-balls

Spicer, Ben, "Children who spend hours glued to their smartphones are more likely to be sleepdeprived and obese" Daily Mail, 14 December 2016, https://www.dailymail.co.uk/health/article-4032434/Children-spend-hours-glued-smartphones-likely-sleep-deprived-obese.html

Williams, Angela, "John Goodman Reveals the Inspiration Behind His Massive Weight Loss," ABC News, 11 Mar 2016, https://abcnews.go.com/Entertainment/john-goodman-reveals-inspiration-massive-weight-loss/story?id=37577068

"'Active' Video Games Burn Calories Study: Kids Who Play Active Video Games Burn Four Times as Many Calories as Kids Who Play Traditional Games," 2 Sept 2008, http:// Children.webmd.com/news/20080902/active-games-burn-calories.

"Burn calories with video games," Consumer Reports on Health, December 2010, https://www.webmd.com/children/news/20080902/active-video-games-burn-calories
"Burn Calories with the Guitar Hero Workout," 13 Dec 2018, https://www.lifewire.com/guitarhero- workout-3562565

"UK Study Finds Significant Health Benefits Associated with Standing," 21 Oct 2013, https://www.prnewswire.com/news-releases/uk-study-finds-significant-health-benefits-associated-with-standing-228616101.html

"Use an Under the desk Exercise Bike to Lose Weight," https://www.weightlossresources.co.uk/exercise/mini-pedal-exerciser-lose-weight.htm

"Female gamers a new risk group for overweight," 24 Sep 2015, https://www.eurekalert.org/pub_releases/2015-09/uog-fga092415.php

"Will Treadmill and Bike Desks Become the New Norm?", https://www.govtech.com/health/Will-Treadmill-Bike-Desks-Become-New-Norm.html